DEEZIFY'S EPIC WORKOUT HANDBOOK

DEEZIFY'S EPIC WORKOUT HANDBOOK

AN ILLUSTRATED GUIDE TO GETTING SWOLE

FIL RUBERTO

TILLER PRESS

NEW YORK LONDON TORONTO SYDNEY NEW DELHI

TILLER PRESS

An Imprint of Simon & Schuster, Inc.
1230 Avenue of the Americas
New York, NY 10020

First Tiller Press trade paperback edition May 2021

TILLER PRESS and colophon are trademarks of Simon & Schuster, Inc.

For information about special discounts for bulk purchases, please contact Simon & Schuster Special Sales at 1-866-506-1949 or business@simonandschuster.com.

The Simon & Schuster Speakers Bureau can bring authors to your live event. For more information or to book an event, contact the Simon & Schuster Speakers Bureau at 1-866-248-3049 or visit our website at www.simonspeakers.com.

Interior design by Matt Ryan

Manufactured in the United States of America

1   3   5   7   9   10   8   6   4   2

Library of Congress Cataloging-in-Publication Data
Names: Ruberto, Fil, author.
Title: Deezify's epic workout handbook : an illustrated guide to getting swole / Fil Ruberto.
Description: New York : Tiller Press, [2021]
Identifiers: LCCN 2020000952 (print) | LCCN 2020000953 (ebook) | ISBN 9781982137410 (paperback) | ISBN 9781982137427 (ebook)
Subjects: LCSH: Exercise. | Physical fitness.
Classification: LCC GV481 .R83 2021 (print) | LCC GV481 (ebook) | DDC 613.7—dc23
LC record available at https://lccn.loc.gov/2020000952
LC ebook record available at https://lccn.loc.gov/2020000953

ISBN 978-1-9821-3741-0
ISBN 978-1-9821-3742-7 (ebook)

CONTENTS

VI INTRODUCTION
X HOW TO USE THIS BOOK

1 THE BODY

3 CHEST
4 Exercises
20 Summary

23 BACK
24 Exercises
41 Summary

45 SHOULDERS
46 Exercises
62 Summary

65 ARMS
66 Biceps Exercises
80 Biceps Summary
82 Triceps Exercises
91 Triceps Summary

93 CORE
94 Exercises
102 Summary

105 LEGS
106 Exercises
131 Summary

135 WORKOUTS OF THE DAY (WODs)

136 Chest God Sacrifice
140 Back Attack
144 Arm-Day Blaster
148 Nine Stages of Hell: Plates
152 Glute Ham Sammich
154 Dread the Sled
156 Back-Beef Basics
157 Leg Killer
158 Crazy Eights
159 Landmine Superset
160 Beyond Delts
161 Planks Pizza Slices (L/R)
162 Valhalla Circuit
163 Big Pipes
164 Yard Work

165 STRETCHES
184 EIGHT-WEEK WORKOUT PLAN
194 GLOSSARY
196 ACKNOWLEDGMENTS

INTRODUCTION

My name is Fil Ruberto, but tens of thousands of people on-line know me as Deezify. What does Deezify mean? Well, it started with the young bros. While I was working out at the gym, they would see me and ask, "Bro, how can I get *deezed* like you?" In case you're unfamiliar (although I can't imagine you are since you're reading this book), "deezed" refers to "diesel," which is slang for "big" or "strong"—much like "swole," "yoked," "jacked," and "pumped."

I have twenty years of natural bodybuilding experience and have been a CANFITPRO Personal Training Specialist, a Fitness Instruc-tor Specialist, and a kettlebell instructor, as well as being certified in ViPR, BOSU, and SMRT (Self-Myofascial Release Technique, also known as foam rolling), but you may be surprised to learn that I haven't always been 240 pounds of muscle. As a kid, I was actually quiet, skinny, and shy, an honor student who liked to draw. At school, you could often catch me outside drawing in my sketchbook while I waited for class to start.

When I graduated from high school in 1993, I won the school's art award and headed to university to pursue a degree in architectural science. Early on in my freshman year, one of my friends started weight lifting. He totally transformed himself, and when I saw his re-sults, I thought, *I can do this.* As someone who grew up being a big comic book fan, who learned to draw by mimicking my favorite art-ists, I decided to apply that same strategy to working out. I've always been motivated and inspired to do things in that way.

My fitness journey began in my garage with some rusty old weights, and the more I worked out with them, the more my passion for fitness grew. For the thesis I had to do in order to complete my architectural-science degree, I even designed a fitness center. Need-less to say, working out had become a big part of my life.

After graduating from university, I worked in the architecture industry for several years, mainly writing health and safety reports for hundreds of commercial buildings, but I eventually began to feel creatively unfulfilled. As a means of addressing this, I taught myself web and graphic design. At the same time, I continued to pursue my passion for fitness. When I turned thirty-five, I had accumulated sixteen years of training myself in the gym, more than ten thousand hours of workouts, and endless hours studying fitness. Training, lifting, working out—whatever you want to call it—started as my hobby. But my hobby then became my habit. Some may even say it became my religion.

I caught the fitness bug young because it physically transformed me and helped me with confidence, so when an opportunity arose to become a certified personal trainer, I seized it, with the goal of being able to use my experience to help others reach their fitness goals. Every personal trainer brings their own past experiences to their training style, and as a former fitness outsider who spent years working in a different industry, I vowed to train people from all walks of life, keep pretentious fitness terminology to a minimum, and always tell my clients the truth. I wanted to be an empathetic and fun trainer, but also stern, like the big brother I am. In other words, there would be no BS in my training—only the promise of hard work ahead.

The idea of workout illustrations came to me when I was planning my first fitness class. I called it the Gladiator Club. While teaching this class, I wanted to stand out from the other instructors, who would simply go through the motions, so I got the idea to run a circuit in order to accommodate the number of people who had signed up for my class. There was one big issue I observed while running the circuits, however: People would not stop asking the question "What is this exercise again?" as they moved to the next station.

I had to come up with a solution, so I decided to sketch out a couple of the exercises to identify them for my clients. I made all the figures in the illustrations gladiators as a nod to the name of the class, and I pinned the drawings on the walls of the studio. This way, every exercise station would be clearly labeled, and class attendees would no longer need to ask what the exercise was.

I could just focus on helping people with their form and offering other guidance. It wasn't long before the class became a hit (with both women and men). After it took off, I started providing clients who were new to lifting with additional sketches that walked them through particular exercises, and I even began designing entirely illustrated exercise programs for a handful of more-experienced clients, so that they could use them when working out on their own.

After training clients for several years, it was time to level up and set another goal, and that goal was to reach more people. As a trainer who had to be in the gym all day, be accessible for walk-ins, abide by gym rules, and work with only gym patrons, I was starting to feel restricted. I liked training people, but I felt like I wasn't reaching everyone I could be reaching, and I also really wanted to focus more on my art. So when I turned forty years old, I decided to make a change. I left the personal-training job and committed to using my technical and creative experience to create something of fitness value that was also motivational. I thought, *If I can produce fitness-oriented artwork that is both entertaining and informative, I'll be killing two dinosaurs with one atlas stone, so to speak.*

That's when I began documenting my knowledge and experiences as a trainer in illustration form for everyone on the Internet—under the name Deezify.

Some people believe you can become an expert at doing something if you practice it for ten thousand hours, and I sure have put in my time doing this. Now that I'm forty-five years old, I want to inspire, motivate, and educate the masses in my own unique way, which leads me to this book.

This is not your ordinary fitness manual. There's plenty of those out there, and most of them consist of either ghostwritten tips from overly photoshopped celebrities or boring, recycled material that's delivered in an uninspiring format. But unlike in those books, in the pages that follow you will find more than one hundred illustrated exercises, custom bodybuilding routines, and an eight-week fitness plan. What's more, a cast of epic and entertaining characters—similar to the gladiators I drew for my clients all those years ago—will guide you through each workout and help you target all areas of your body.

Learning never stops. Those who assume they know everything are doomed. So become a sponge. Today I'm bigger, stronger, and smarter than I was twenty years ago because of this mentality. Ultimately, my goal with this book is to feed your passion for fitness, help you transform your body, and encourage you to keep going. If I can make you smile while doing so, that's pretty good, too.

—FIL (DEEZIFY)

HOW TO USE THIS BOOK

This handbook contains a collection of illustrated exercises, workout routines, and stretches, complete with step-by-step instructions, that will help you take your fitness regimen to the next level. While you may need to familiarize yourself with some terminology before you can perform these exercises (flip to the back of the book for a helpful glossary), you won't find any difficult-to-understand kinesiology or anatomy terms in this book like you would find in other fitness manuals. In my experience working with clients from different backgrounds, jargony words can often be off-putting or intimidating, so I've made a point to not regurgitate a bunch of them here.

The instructions for every exercise, workout routine, and stretch are relatively simple and to the point. All of them are accompanied by easy-to-read text and descriptive illustrations that show you exactly how an exercise should be done. On every exercise, workout routine, and stretch page, you will find the name of the move or routine, the equipment needed, the number of sets and repetitions you should complete, the tempo (if applicable), the amount of time you should rest between sets, and any additional information you should be mindful of when performing certain exercises.

The exercises in the Body section have been grouped into chapters according to the major areas of the body you'll be targeting, and within each chapter the exercises are further organized by equipment (such as barbells or dumbbells) and rated according to level of difficulty by a series of stars shown at the bottom of the page. The greater the number of shaded-in stars, the more difficult or demanding the exercise or workout is. At the end of each chapter, you will also find a summary of the section that contains additional notes, modifications (abbreviated as MOD), and exercise adjustments or routine variations (noted as SETS). I've done this to keep the individual exercise pages clean and brief, as well as to provide a simple referencing system for you at the end of each chapter.

The Workouts of the Day (or WODs) section is a collection of some of my favorite workout routines. They are a mix of body part–specific splits (workouts divided by muscle groups), circuits, and specialty workouts, and they feature step-by-step illustrations as well as helpful annotations.

Similarly, the Stretches section of this book is a collection of post-workout static stretches with accompanying instructions. These stretches can be done daily as part of your flexibility training or post-workout recovery. Stretching is incredibly important because it aids muscle recovery, reduces muscle tension from workouts, and reduces injury during workouts. It also improves performance in daily activities, workouts, and sports.

Feel free to perform the exercises or workouts individually, or use them to customize your own routine. If you're looking for more guidance than that, however, I've also included an Eight-Week Workout Plan toward the end of the book that you can use to jump-start your physical transformation.

Because I can only be your virtual coach, it's impossible for me to correct your form when you're performing these exercises and routines, just as I also can't hold you accountable for your work and commitment. So I encourage you to consult a certified personal trainer in order to learn proper exercise techniques and protocols, as well as to consult your physician, which you should do before starting any exercise program—especially if you are a beginner. Also, it's important to remember: Soreness is good, pain is bad. If you are experiencing any pain when doing these exercises, workout routines, and stretches, then stop what you're doing immediately.

Finally, this is not an end-all-be-all fitness manual. It is simply a fun and unique handbook designed to inspire, motivate, and educate you on your fitness journey. And just as many heroes have had the help of a guide who shares their knowledge and motivates the hero to overcome obstacles, I am here to be yours.

It's time for you to be the hero. So let's begin, my friend.

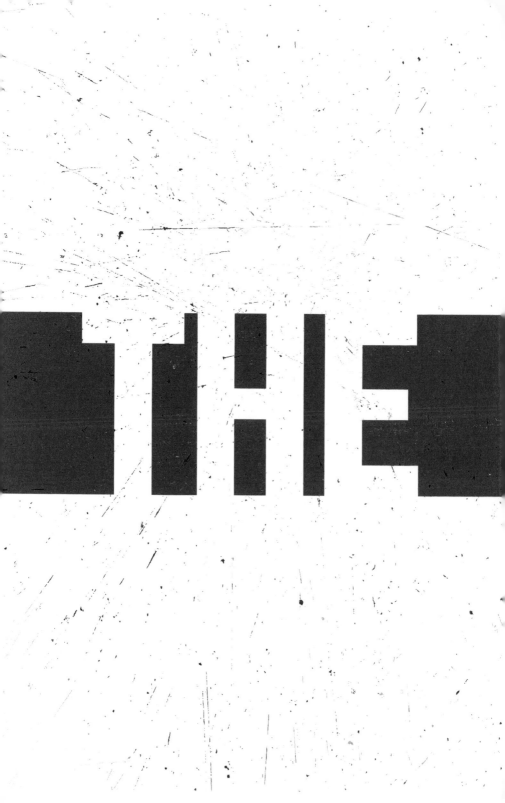

BODY

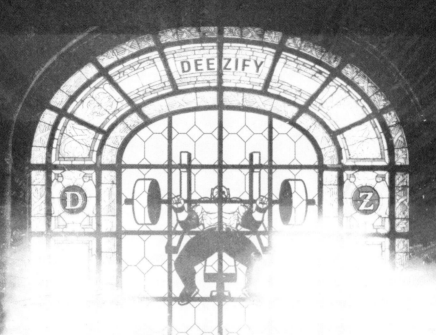

WHEN MY SAVAGE
LORD WAS ASKED
HOW MANY MORE SETS
ON BENCH HE HAD LEFT,
HE REPLIED,
"ALL OF THEM."

PECTORALIS

CHEST

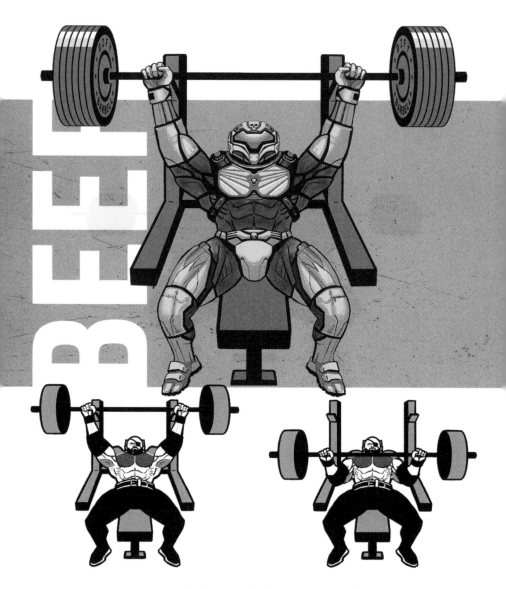

BARBELL BENCH PRESS
3 sets x 3 reps (90% 1RM) - rest 120s

TIP: Warm up and build up appropriately.
Max 5 reps/set if pyramiding up.

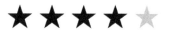

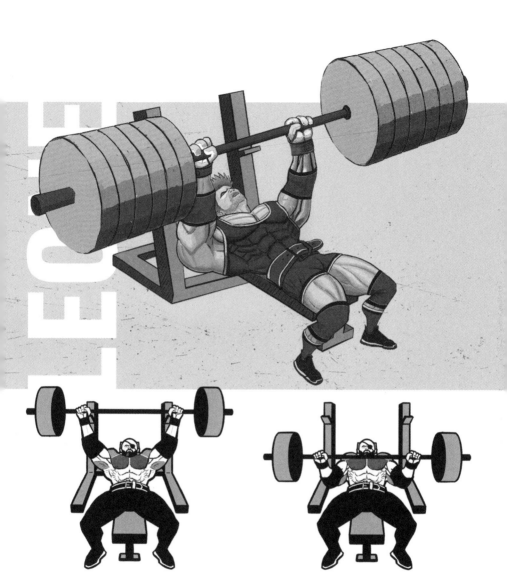

BARBELL BENCH PRESS
4 sets x 10 reps (70% 1RM) - rest 60s

TIP: All 4 sets should be done at the same weight
(70% 1RM). Warm up appropriately.

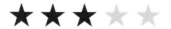

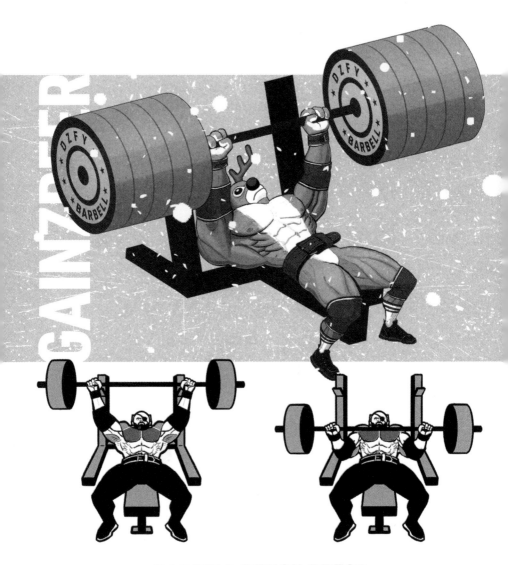

BARBELL BENCH PRESS
5 sets x 5 reps (80% 1RM) - rest 90s

TIP: Build up appropriately.
Max 5 reps/set if pyramiding up.

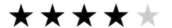

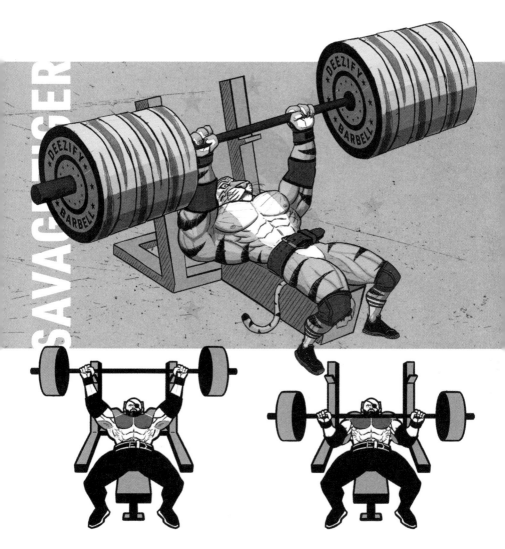

BARBELL BENCH PRESS–1½ REPS
4 sets x 8 reps - rest 60s
(1 rep = 1 full + bottom ½ rep)

TIP: The bar should tap the chest.

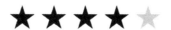

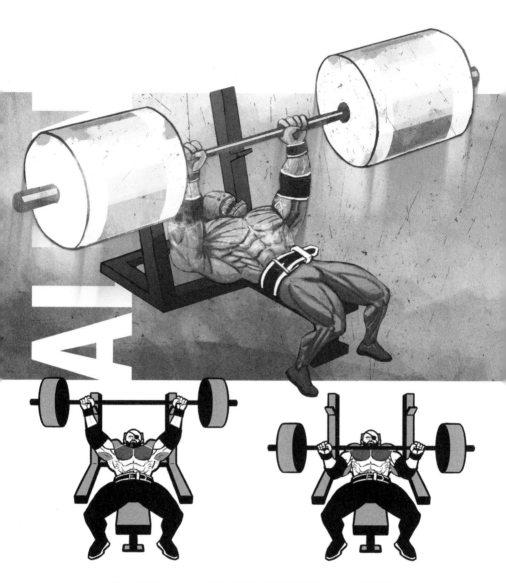

BARBELL BENCH PRESS–SPEED
8 sets x 3 reps (30% 1RM) - rest 60s

TIP: Reps should be explosive.
Remember: less weight, less reps, more speed.

★ ★ ★ ☆ ☆

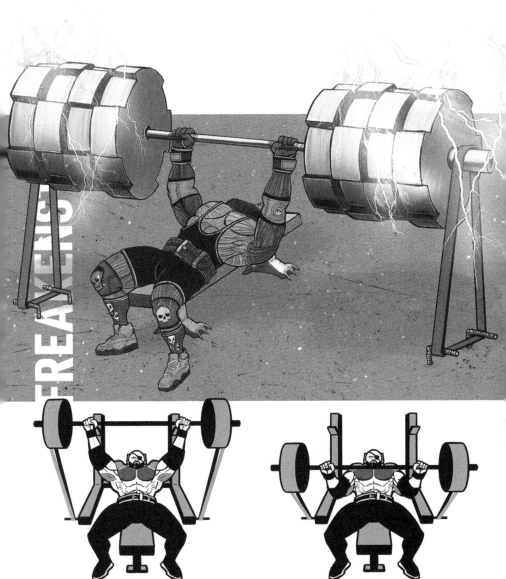

BARBELL BENCH PRESS WITH BANDS
6 sets x 5 reps - rest 60s
(PR band tension: 40% bottom, 70% top)

TIP: Build up appropriately.

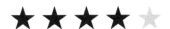

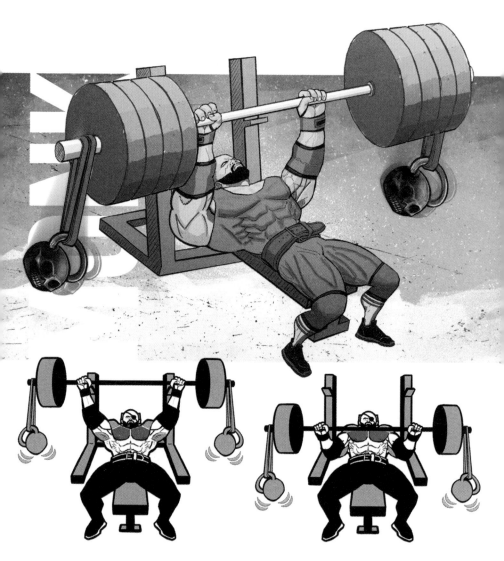

BARBELL BENCH–BAND-SUSPENDED WEIGHTS

5 sets x 8 reps (2210) - rest 60s

(2s lower - 2s pause - 1s press - 0)

TIP: Suspend kettlebells or plates.

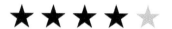

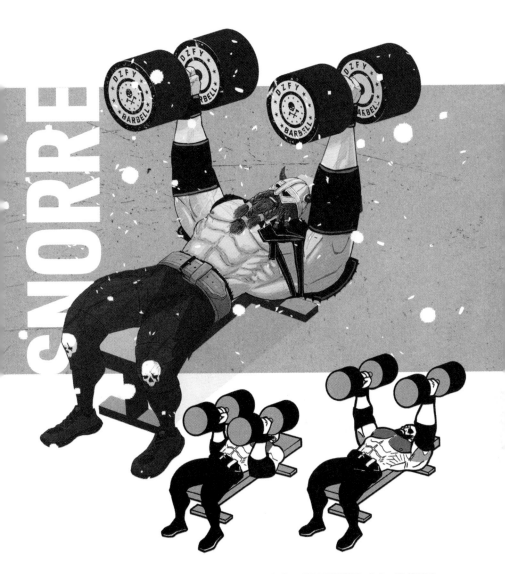

DUMBBELL CHEST PRESS—NEUTRAL GRIP
5 sets x 10 reps - rest 60s

TIP: 10 reps should be difficult. Use a neutral grip
(i.e., palms should be facing each other) or standard press.

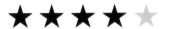

★ ★ ★ ★ ☆

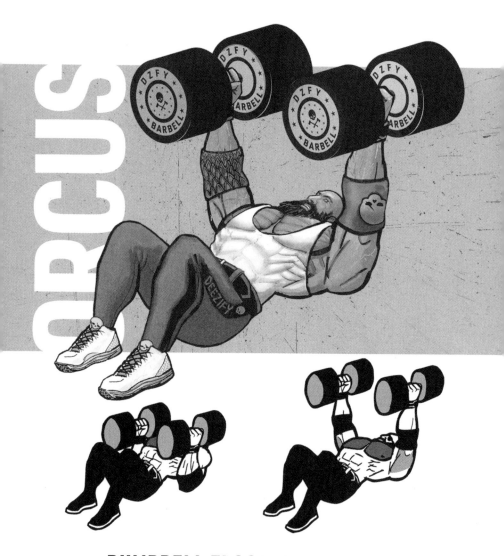

DUMBBELL FLOOR-CHEST PRESS
4 sets x 8 reps (2010) - rest 60s

(2s lower - 0 - 1s press - 0)

TIP: This is a shoulder-friendly chest press.

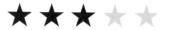

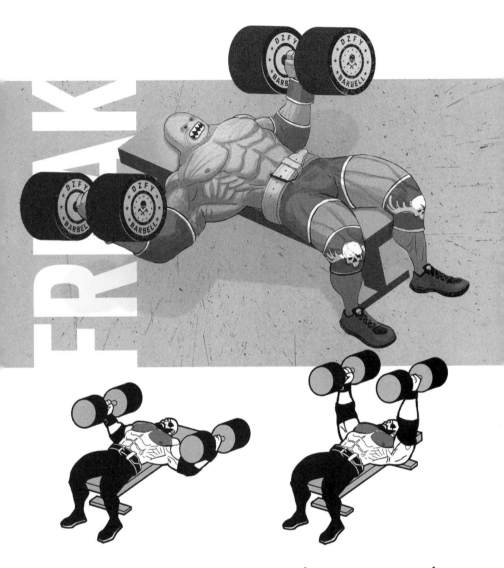

DUMBBELL CHEST FLYES (RUN RACK UP)
6+ sets x 8 reps (2010) - rest 45s
(2s lower - 0 - 1s flye - 0)

TIP: To pyramid up, add 5–10 lbs/set.

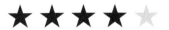

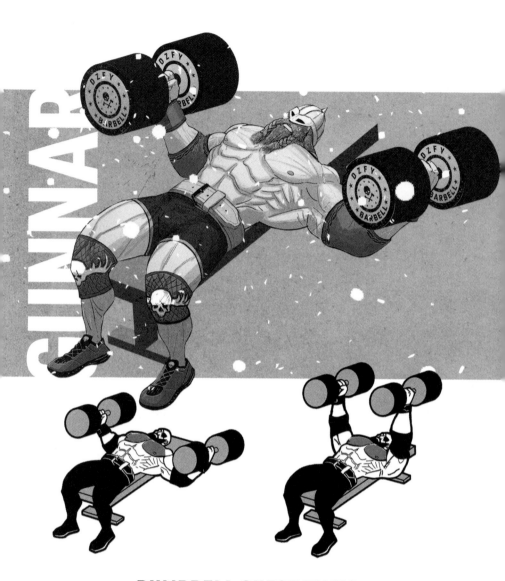

DUMBBELL CHEST FLYES
4 sets x 8 reps (3010) - rest 60s
(3s lower - 0 - 1s flye - 0)

TIP: Build up appropriately.

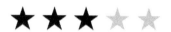

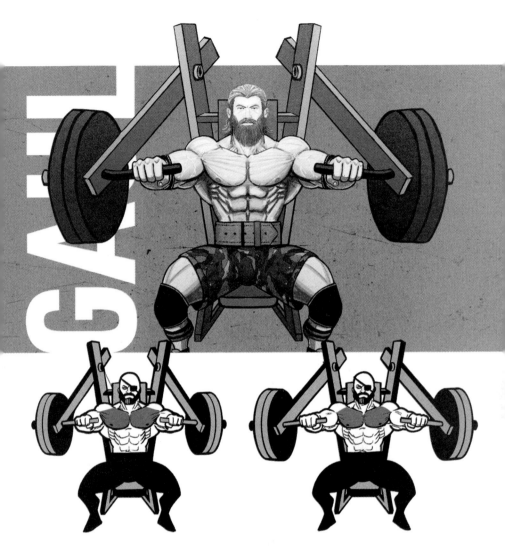

MACHINE CHEST PRESS (DIRTY 30s)
4 sets x 10, 10, 10 reps - rest 60s
(10 top ½, 10 bottom ½, 10 full reps)

TIP: Applicable on any chest machine.

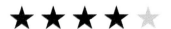

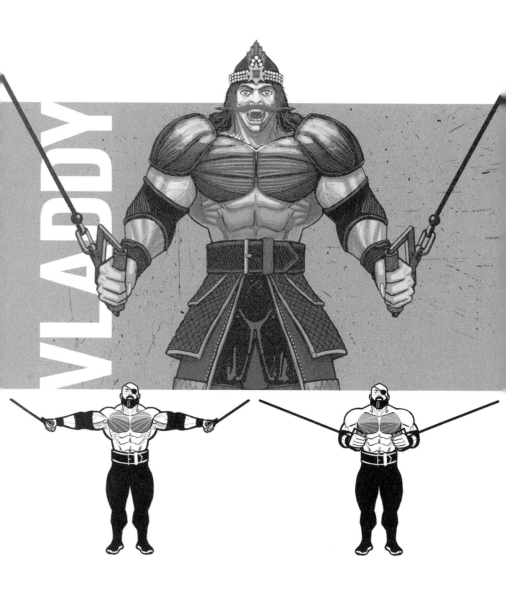

CABLE/HANDLE CHEST FLYES–LOW

4 sets x 8 reps (2010) - rest 45s

(2s lower - 0 - 1s flye - 0)

TIP: Flye toward your lower pecs.

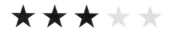

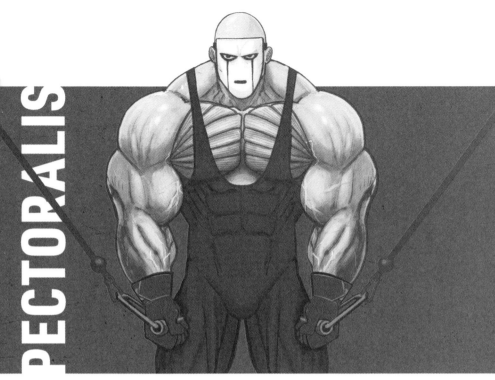

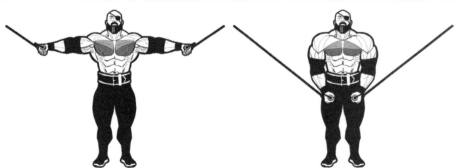

CABLE/HANDLE CHEST FLYES–VERTICAL
4 sets x 8 reps (2012) - rest 60s
(2s lower - 0 - 1s flye - 2s squeeze)

TIP: Vertical flye toward your upper thighs.

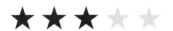

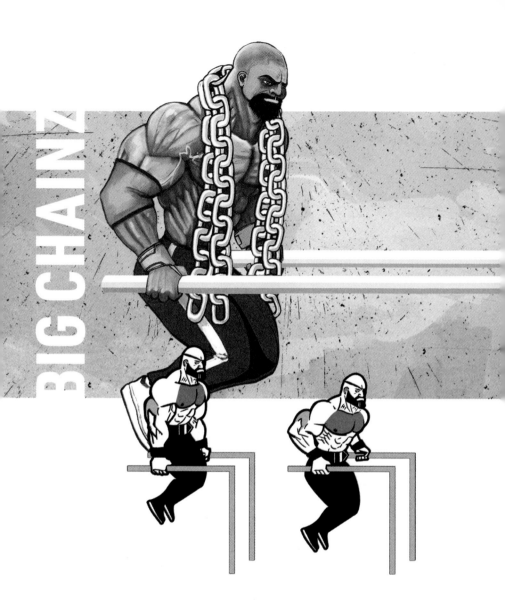

BIG CHAINZ

CHAIN-WEIGHTED CHEST DIPS
4 sets x 10 reps or until failure - rest 60s

TIP: Build up with more chains (or weight) until 10 reps are difficult to complete. Lean forward for chest emphasis.

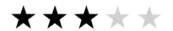

MORTAL MEN DO PUSH UPS, SAVAGES DO EARTH DOWNS. CHANGE YOUR PERSPECTIVE.

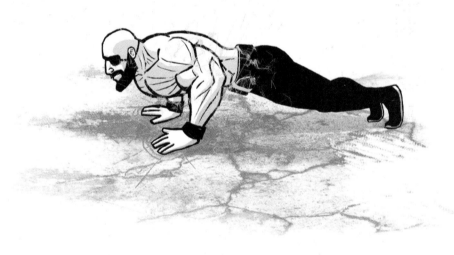

~~PUSH-UPS~~ EARTH-DOWNS
100 total reps - rest when needed

TIP: Complete in the least amount of time possible.
Add chains for more resistance.

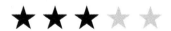

CHEST EXERCISES SUMMARY

BARBELL BENCH PRESS
3 sets x 3 reps (90% 1RM) - rest 120s

BARBELL BENCH PRESS
4 sets x 10 reps (70% 1RM) - rest 60s

BARBELL BENCH PRESS
5 sets x 5 reps (80% 1RM) - rest 90s

MOD
· Adjust hand positions for variety.
  Go wider for the outside of the
  chest, closer for the triceps.

SETS
· **Power:** 3 sets x 3 reps
  (90% 1RM) - rest 120s
· **Strength:** 5 sets x 8 reps - rest 60s
· **Strength:** 4 sets x 8 reps (3010) - rest 60s

BARBELL BENCH PRESS–1½ REPS
4 sets x 8 reps - rest 60s
· 1 rep = 1 full + bottom ½ rep
· The extra ½ rep at the bottom is the
  most difficult part of the press because
  it's more work at the bottom.

MOD
· **Machine Chest Presses:** can be
  implemented on other exercises.

SET
· **Strength:** 3 sets x 10 reps - rest 60s

BARBELL BENCH PRESS–SPEED
8 sets x 3 reps (30% 1RM) - rest 60s
· Speed Bench is pressing the bar as
  explosively as possible. It's less reps,
  less weight, and more speed.

MOD
· Add pause at the bottom,
  and press explosively.

SET
· **Speed:** 8 sets x 2 reps
  (40% 1RM) - rest 60s

BARBELL BENCH PRESS WITH BANDS
6 sets x 5 reps - rest 60s - PR band
tension: 40% bottom, 70% top

MOD
· Adjust bands for appropriate tightness.

SET
· **Power:** 3 sets x 3 reps - rest 120s
· **Power:** 5 sets x 5 reps - rest 90s
· **Strength:** 4 sets x 8 reps - rest 60s

BARBELL BENCH–BAND-SUSPENDED WEIGHTS
5 sets x 8 reps (2210) - rest 60s
· (2s lower - 2s pause - 1s press - 0)

MOD
· Suspend kettlebells or plates/suspend
  multiple bands on each side.

SET
· **Strength:** 4 sets x 6 reps - rest 60s
· **Strength:** 3 sets x 10 reps - rest 60s

DUMBBELL CHEST PRESS–NEUTRAL GRIP
5 sets x 10 reps - rest 60s

MOD
· Dumbbell Incline Chest
  Press 30–15 degrees

SET
· **Pyramid Up:** 3 sets x 10 reps - rest 60s -
  increase 10 lbs/set to 3 working sets
· **Power:** 5 sets x 8 reps - rest 60s

SUPERSET WITH CHEST FLYES
· **Warm Up:** 5 sets x 20 reps

DUMBBELL FLOOR-CHEST PRESS
4 sets x 8 reps (2010) - rest 60s
· (2s lower - 0 - 1s press - 0)
· Floor presses are more shoulder-friendly because your shoulders are supported by the floor.

MOD
· Dumbbell Single-Arm Floor Press/ Barbell Floor-Chest Press

SET
· **Strength:** 4 sets x 10 reps - rest 60s
· **Strength:** 5 sets x 8 reps - rest 60s

DUMBBELL CHEST FLYES (RUN RACK UP)
6+ sets x 8 reps (2010) - rest 45s
· (2s lower - 0 - 1s flye - 0)
· To pyramid up, use 5–10 lbs/set.

DUMBBELL CHEST FLYES
4 sets x 8 reps (3010) - rest 60s
· (3s lower - 0 - 1s flye - 0)

MOD
· DB Incline Chest Flyes 30–15 degrees

SET
· **Strength:** 4 sets x 10 reps - rest 60s
· **Strength:** 5 sets x 8 reps - rest 60s

MACHINE CHEST PRESS (DIRTY 30s)
4 sets x 10, 10, 10 reps - rest 60s
· 10 top ½, 10 bottom ½, 10 full reps

MOD
· Machine Chest Presses at different angles (incline or decline) and hand positions (close or wide).
· Single-Arm or Two-Arm Chest Presses

SET
· **Strength:** 4 sets x 10 reps - rest 60s
· **Strength:** 5 sets x 8 reps - rest 60s
· **Warm Up:** 5 sets x 20 reps (40%)

CABLE/HANDLE CHEST FLYES—LOW
4 sets x 8 reps (2010) - rest 45s
· (2s lower - 0 - 1s flye - 0)

CABLE/HANDLE CHEST FLYES—VERTICAL
4 sets x 8 reps (2012) - rest 60s
· (2s lower - 0 - 1s flye - 2s squeeze)

MOD
· Flye at different angles for full pec development.

SET
· 3 sets x 10 reps - rest 45s
· 4 sets x 8 reps - rest 45s
· **Compound set:** Cable Chest Flyes Vertical, Low, and Bent Over

CHAIN-WEIGHTED CHEST DIPS
4 sets x 10 reps or until failure - rest 60s
· Lean forward for chest emphasis. Add weight when regular dips are easy.

MOD
· Add weight via chains, weighted belt, or weighted vest.
· Time under tension: Slow down your reps.

SET
· 4 sets x 6 reps.
· (5s lower - 0 - 1s lift - 0) - rest 60s

~~PUSH-UPS~~ EARTH-DOWNS
100 total reps - rest when needed
· Complete in the least amount of time possible.

MOD
· Add chains for more resistance.

SET
· 4 sets x 25 reps - rest 45s
· **Warm-up:** 5 sets x 20 reps

BETTER TO GO BACK THAN TO GO WRONG

BACK

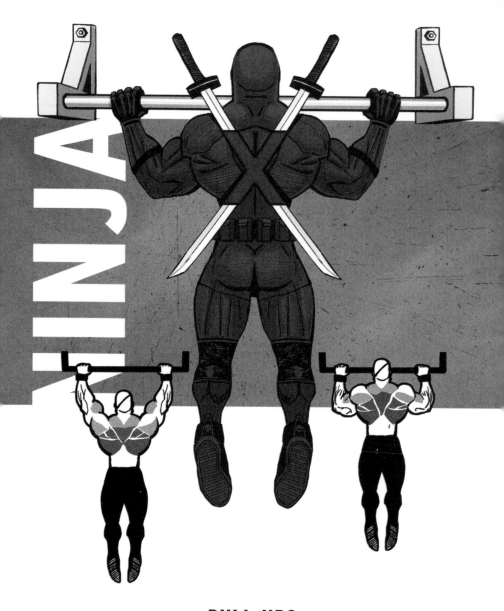

NINJA

PULL-UPS
100 total reps

TIP: Perform as many reps as possible per set.
Rest as long as you like.

★★★★☆

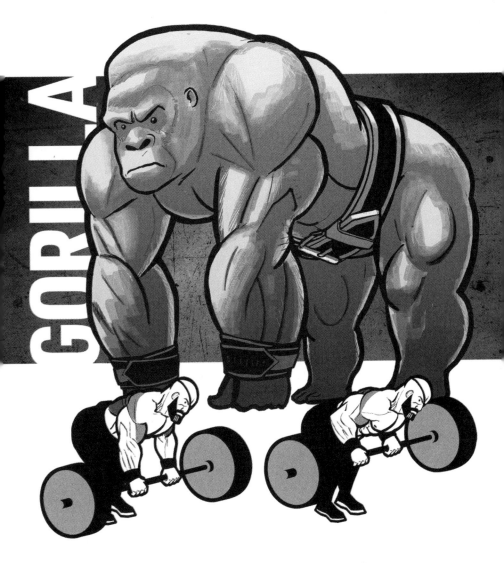

BARBELL PENDLAY ROWS
5 sets x 5 reps (80% 1RM) - rest 90s

TIP: Each rep must start from the floor.
Keep the back parallel to the ground.

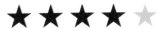

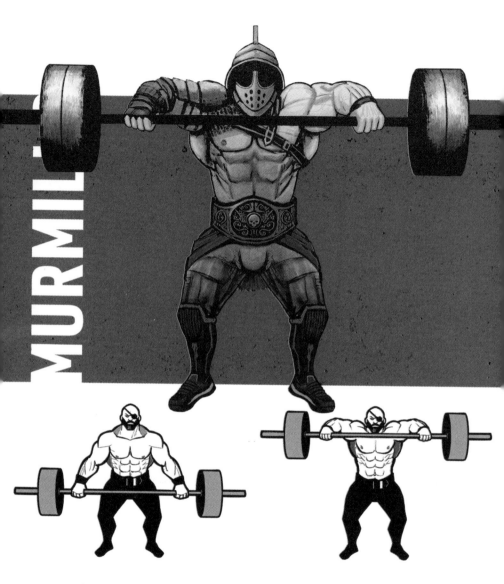

MURMIL

BARBELL HIGH-PULLS SNATCH GRIP
5 sets x 6 reps - rest 60s

TIP: Use a wider snatch grip.
Generate power through the hips.

★ ★ ★ ★ ☆

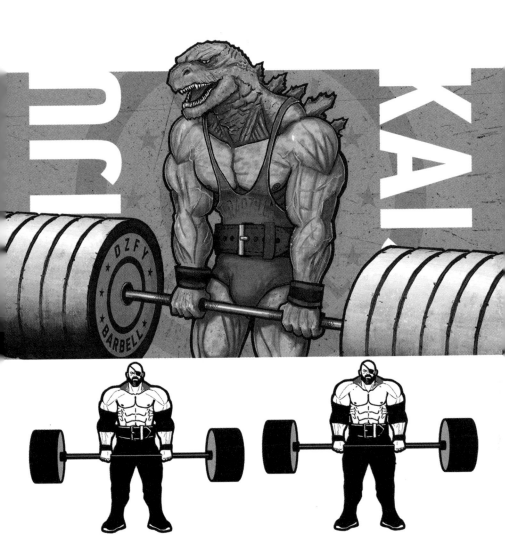

BARBELL SHRUGS (PYRAMID UP)
5 reps/set to max - rest 60s
(Build up using 25- and 45-lb plates only.)

TIP: Use strict form. No knee-bending.

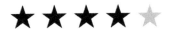

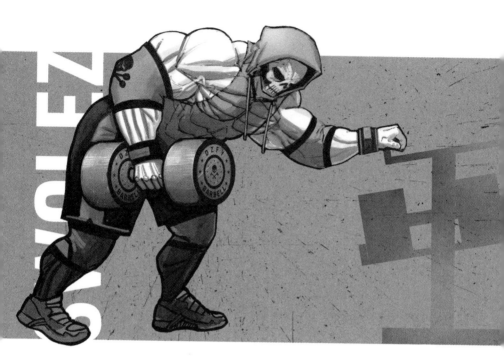

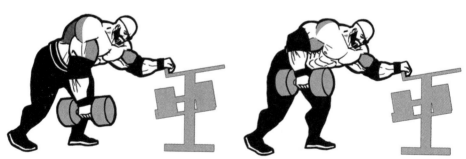

DUMBBELL BENT-OVER ROWS
(L/R; RUN RACK UP)
6± sets x 6 reps - rest 45s

(+10 lbs/set to 3 sets x 6 reps max)

TIP: Keep the back parallel to the ground.

★ ★ ★ ★ ☆

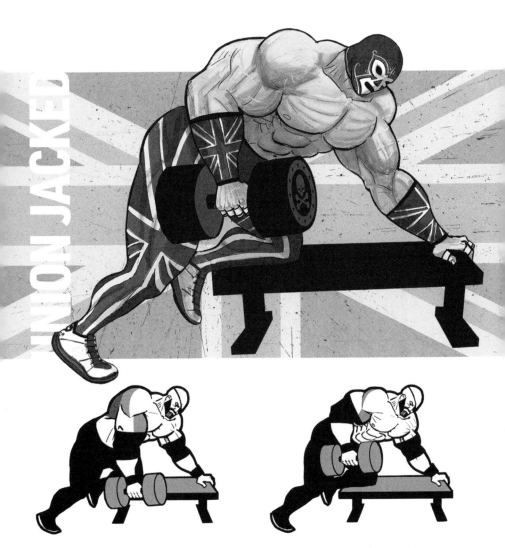

DUMBBELL BENT-OVER ROWS (L/R)
5 sets x 10 reps (2010) - rest 45s
(2s lower - 0 - 1s row - 0)

TIP: Keep the back parallel to the floor.

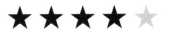

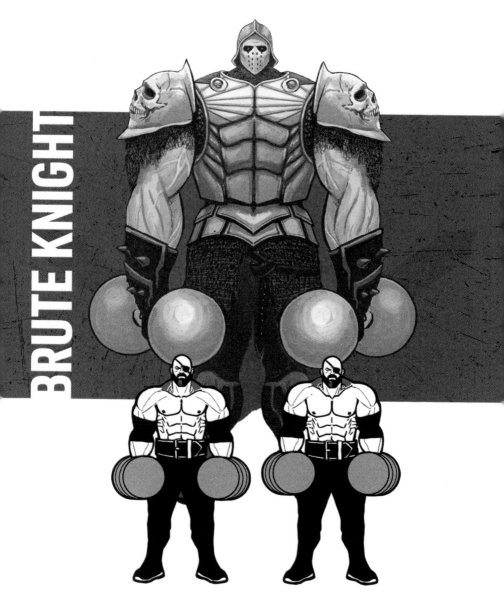

BRUTE KNIGHT

DUMBBELL SHRUGS
4 sets x 10 reps (2011) - rest 60s
(2s lower - 0 - 1s shrug - 1s top hold)

TIP: No lifting straps for grip strength.

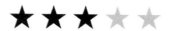

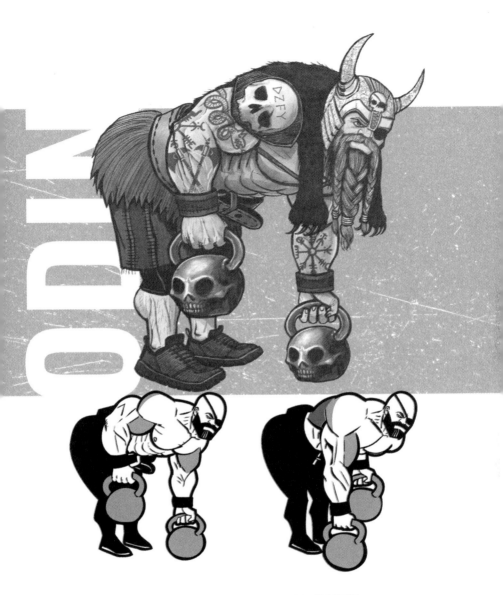

KETTLEBELL BENT-OVER ALTERNATING ROWS
4 sets x 20 reps - rest 45s

TIP: Keep the back parallel to the ground.

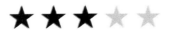

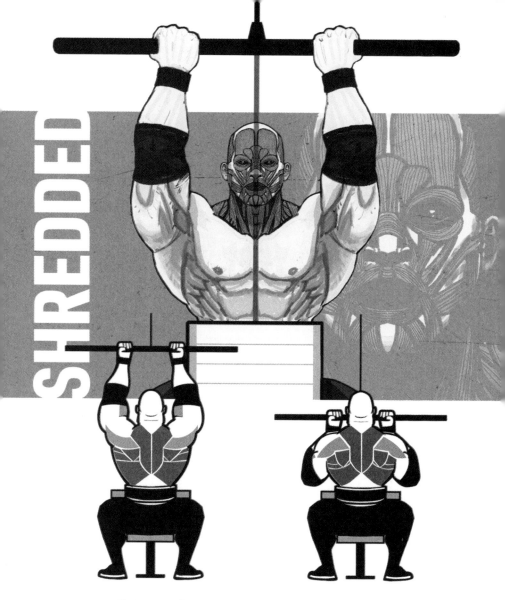

CABLE/BAR LAT PULL-DOWNS
4 sets x 8 reps (3010) - rest 45s
(3s lower - 0 - 1s pull-down - 0)

TIP: Use a palm-up grip. Pull down to the chin.

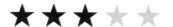

★ ★ ★ ☆ ☆

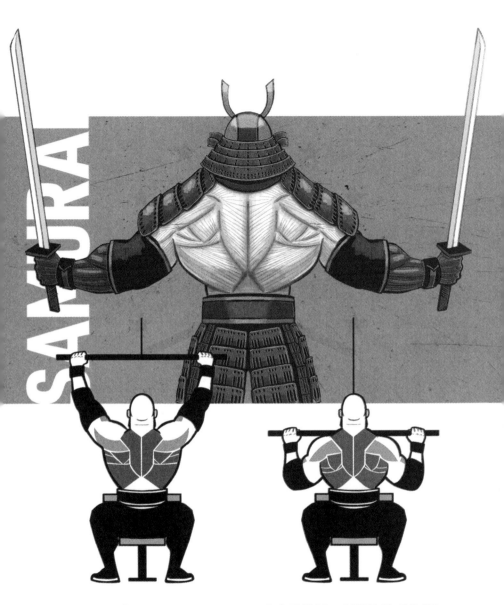

SAMURAI

CABLE/BAR LAT PULL-DOWNS—WIDE GRIP
10-2 reps run rack up - rest 45s
(Start at 40%; increase 1 pin/set.)

TIP: Grip the bar a bit wider than shoulder-width.

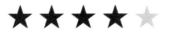

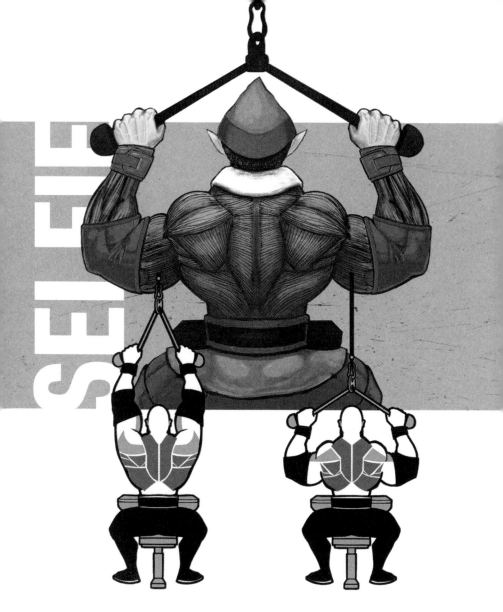

CABLE/ROPE PULL-DOWNS
4 sets x 10 reps (3010) - rest 45s
(3s lower - 0 - 1s pull-down - 0)

TIP: Pull the rope apart while lowering.

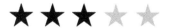

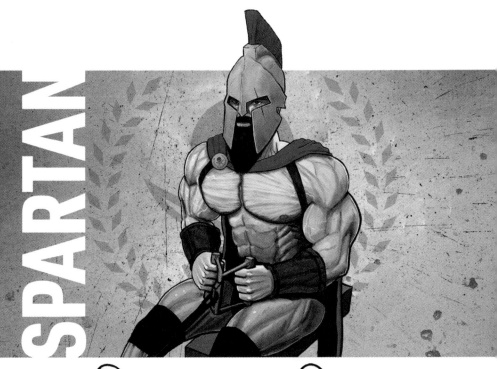

SPARTAN

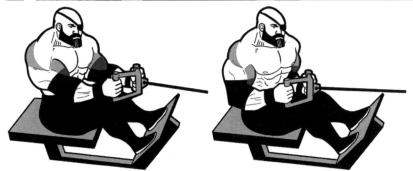

CABLE/V-HANDLE SEATED LAT ROWS

10 reps - rest 10s; 20 reps - rest 20s; 30 reps - rest 30s; 40 reps (40% 1RM)

TIP: Pull toward the upper abs.

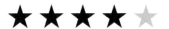

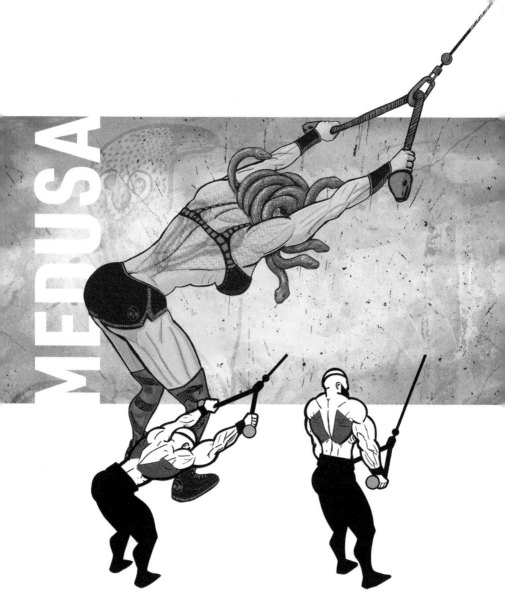

CABLE/ROPE LAT PUSH-DOWNS
4 sets x 8 reps + drop set (3010) - rest 45s
(3s lower - 0 - 1s push-down - 0)

Drop set = reduce 20%/set
100%, 80%, 60%, and then 40%.

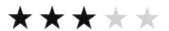

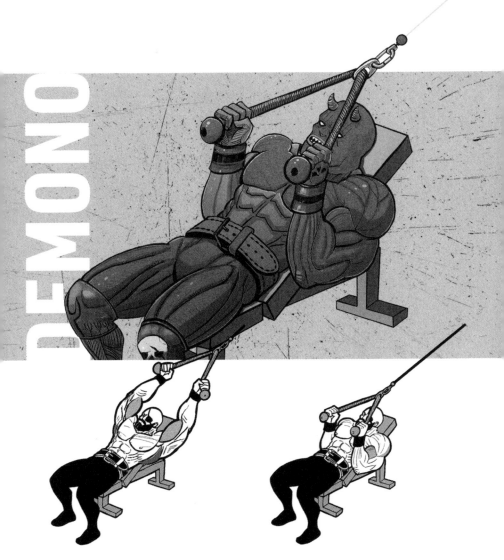

DEMONO

CABLE/ROPE INCLINE LAT PULL-DOWNS
4 sets x 8 reps (3010) - rest 45s
(3s lower - 0 - 1s pull-down - 0)

TIP: Pull through and stop at the chest.

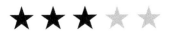

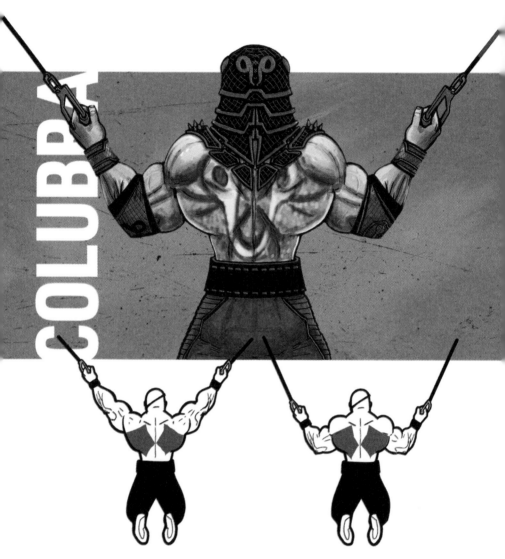

CABLE KNEELING LAT "W" PULL-DOWNS
4 sets x 8 reps (3011) - rest 45s
(3s lower - 0 - 1s pull-down - 1s hold)

TIP: Kneel or sit on the bench.

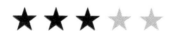

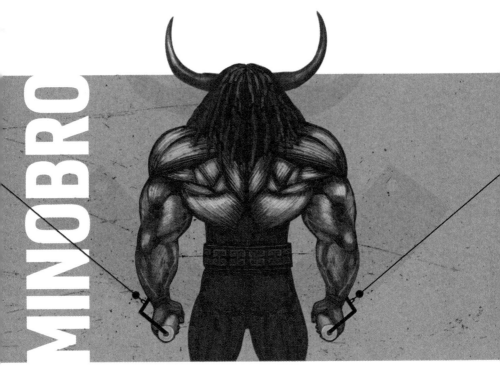

MINOBRO

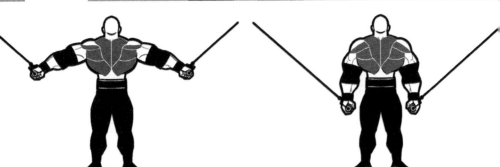

CABLE/HANDLE LAT FLYES
4 sets x 10 reps (3010) - rest 45s

(3s lower - 0 - 1s flye - 0)

TIP: Pull handles toward the glutes.

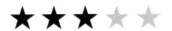

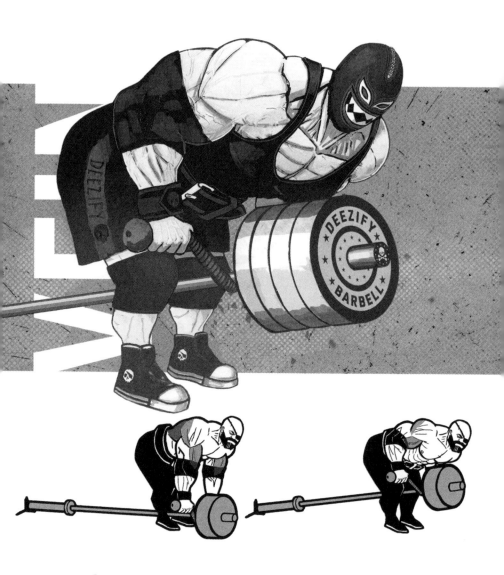

LANDMINE/ROPE BENT-OVER ROWS
4 sets x 5 reps - rest 60s

TIP: Tap each rep on the ground.
Use V-handle for alternative grip.

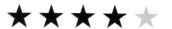

★ ★ ★ ★ ☆

BACK EXERCISES SUMMARY

PULL-UPS
100 total reps
· Pull-ups are performed with a pronated (overhand) grip that's a bit wider than shoulder-width. Keep your chin up, and try to pull your chin to your hands. Don't swing and cheat with your lower body.

MOD
· Chin-ups are performed with a supinated (underhand) grip. Mix up your grip.
· **Regression:** Negative-only pull-ups.
  · Step up into the contracted pull-up position, and slowly lower yourself for the rep. Eventually you will be able to perform a complete rep.
  · **# of reps:** beginners, 30 total; intermediate, 50 total; advanced, 100 total reps.
  · For advanced, add a weight belt or use a slower rep tempo.

SET
· AMRAP/set for 100 reps total
· **Pull-ups for time:** Complete as many reps as you can in 10 minutes.
· 5 reps/set - rest 30s

BARBELL PENDLAY ROWS
5 sets x 5 reps (80% 1RM) - rest 90s
· Each rep must start from the floor, and each rep dies on the floor. Keep your back parallel to the ground. Come to a complete dead stop. Repeat. I recommend using 45-pound plates or bumper plates for proper setup.

SET
· **Power:** 3 sets x 3 reps; 5, 5, 3, 3, 1, 1 reps - rest 90s
· **Hypertrophy:** 5 sets x 5 reps - rest 60s
· **Strength:** 4 sets x 8 reps - rest 45s

BARBELL HIGH-PULLS SNATCH GRIP
5 sets x 6 reps - rest 60s
· A wider snatch grip will create more back engagement. The movement is not an upright row. Shoulders are not involved with the lift.

SET
· **Power:** 3 sets x 3 reps; 5 sets x 5 reps
· **Hypertrophy:** 4 sets x 8 reps

BARBELL SHRUGS (PYRAMID UP)
5 reps/set to max - rest 60s
· Grip the bar, and lift only with your traps. Drive your traps to your ears.

MOD
· **Equipment variation:** Machine shrugs or plate-loaded machine shrugs.
· Use lifting straps for back focus. Don't use straps for grip strength.

SET
· **Power/Strength:** 5 sets x 5 reps
· **Hypertrophy:** 4 sets x 10 reps; 5 sets x 8 reps
· **Drop set:** 100%, 80%, 60%, and then 40%.

DUMBBELL BENT-OVER ROWS (L/R; RUN RACK UP)
6± sets x 6 reps - rest 45s
· A simple way to keep the back parallel to the ground is to tap the dumbbell on the ground with each rep.

SET
· **Heavy:** 5 sets x 10 reps - rest 60s

DUMBBELL BENT-OVER ROWS (L/R)

5 sets x 10 reps (2010) - rest 45s
- (2s lower - 0 - 1s row - 0)
- Take a staggered position on the bench. One extended arm supports the upper body on the bench, while the opposite leg is positioned on the floor. Keep the back parallel to the floor.

SET
- **Strength:** 5 sets x 8 reps - rest 60s
- **Endurance:** 4 sets x 12 reps - rest 60s

DUMBBELL SHRUGS

4 sets x 10 reps (2011) - rest 60s
- (2s lower - 0 - 1s shrug - 1s top hold)

MOD
- Perform standing or seated on the bench with dumbbells to the side.

SET
- **Heavy:** 5 sets x 10 reps - rest 60s - choose heaviest dumbbells
- **Hypertrophy:** 5 sets x 20 reps - heavy dumbbells
- **Iso hold:** 4 sets x 10 reps + 20s contraction at the top

KETTLEBELL BENT-OVER ALTERNATING ROWS

4 sets x 20 reps - rest 45s
- Bend over with both kettlebells on ground. Lift one kettlebell in a row movement while the other kettlebell stays static on the ground. Lower the kettlebell and rest it on the ground. Repeat with the other arm in alternating row fashion.

MOD
- Can substitute with dumbbells.
- **Varying movements:** double rows, isometric hold at top, or single-arm rows.

SET
- 3 sets x 8 reps (3010) - 3s lower - rest 60s

CABLE/BAR LAT PULL-DOWNS

4 sets x 8 reps (3010) - rest 45s
- (3s lower - 0 - 1s pull-down - 0)

MOD
- Vary with bars, V-handle, or double handles.
- Machine Lat Pulldowns, double-arm or single-arm.

SET
- **Run stack up:** 8 reps/set - start at 40% RM and increase weight 1 pin/set

CABLE/BAR LAT PULL-DOWNS—WIDE GRIP

10-2 reps run rack up - rest 45s

MOD
- Vary with bars or a neutral grip bar.
- Machine Lat Pull-Downs, double-arm or single-arm.

SET
- **Hypertrophy:** 4 sets x 8 reps (4010) - rest 45s
- **Strength:** 4 sets x 8-6 reps - rest 45s

CABLE/ROPE PULL-DOWNS

4 sets x 10 reps (3010) - rest 45s
- (3s lower - 0 - 1s pull-down - 0)
- Try to pull the rope apart as you pull down. While lowering, try to keep the rope pulled apart to engage your traps.

MOD
- Attach double handles, and try to pull the handles apart.
- Lean back 15 degrees for back-angle variation.

SET
- **Basic:** 4 sets x 10 reps
- **Dirty 30s:** 3 sets x 10, 10, 10 reps (to eyes, to neck, to chest)

CABLE/V-HANDLE SEATED LAT ROWS

10 reps - rest 10s; 20 reps - rest 20s;
30 reps - rest 30s; 40 reps (40% 1RM)

MOD
- **Equipment variation:** Use V-handle, 2 handles, straight bar, Lat Row Machines.
- Rows toward belly button, rows toward chest, single-arm handle rows.

SET
- **Basic:** 3 sets x 10 reps
- **Heavy:** 4 sets x 8 reps; 5 sets x 5 reps

CABLE/ROPE LAT PUSH-DOWNS

4 sets x 8 reps + drop set (3010) - rest 45s
- (3s lower - 0 - 1s push-down - 0)

MOD
- Use rope or straight bar.

SET
- **Strength:** 3 sets x 10 reps
- **Superset:** Kayak Rows, Seated Rows, or Pull-Ups

CABLE/ROPE INCLINE LAT PULL-DOWNS

4 sets x 8 reps (3010) - rest 45s
- (3s lower - 0 - 1s pull-down - 0)
- Position an incline bench against a cable-machine vertical bar. Adjust the incline bench angle to approximately 60 degrees.

MOD
- Handle Single-Arm Lat Pull-Downs (L/R)

SET
- **Basic:** 3 sets x 10 reps; 4 sets x 10 reps

CABLE KNEELING LAT "W" PULL-DOWNS

4 sets x 8 reps (3011) - rest 45s
- (3s lower - 0 - 1s pull-down - 1s hold)
- Grab handles and kneel on the floor to perform the exercise. Placing a mat or half-foam roller on the floor will make this easier on the knees, or you can sit on a bench or plyo box.

SET
- **Basic:** 4 sets x 10 reps - rest 45s. Change tempos and add contraction hold.
- **Pyramid Up:** 5 sets x 10–6 reps - rest 45s

CABLE/HANDLE LAT FLYES

4 sets x 10 reps (3010) - rest 45s
- (3s lower - 0 - 1s flye - 0)
- Use lighter weight and engage your back, keeping strict form.

SET
- 4 sets x 10 reps - rest 45s
- Superset with Cable Chest Flyes

LANDMINE/ROPE BENT-OVER ROWS

4 sets x 5 reps - rest 60s
- Keep back parallel to the ground. Tap the ground with each rep. For more range of motion, use 25-lb plates instead of 45-lb plates.

MOD
- Use a V-handle or landmine bar for an easier grip instead of rope.
- T-Bar Row Machine

SET
- **Basic:** 4 sets x 8 reps - rest 45s
- **Power:** 5 sets x 5 reps; 5, 5, 3, 3, 3 reps

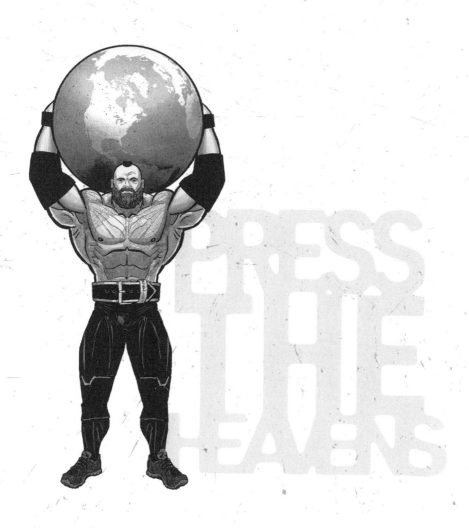

SHOULDERS

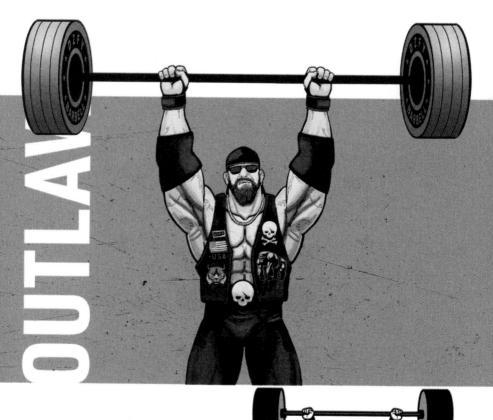

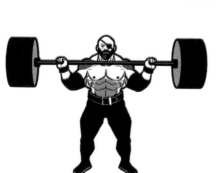 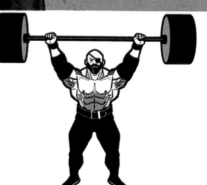

BARBELL SHOULDER PRESS
3 sets x 8 reps - rest 60s

TIP: Build up to 3 working sets.
Maintain strict style. Don't use your hips.

★ ★ ★ ★ ☆

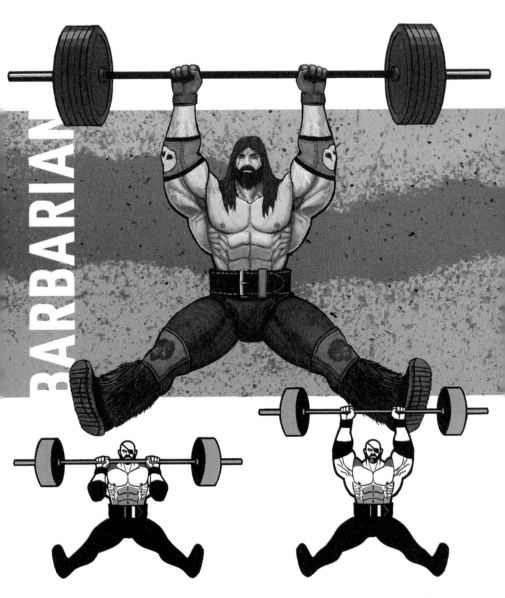

BARBARIAN

BARBELL FLOOR-SEATED SHOULDER PRESS
4 sets x 8 reps - rest 60s

TIP: Perform press in power rack.
Keep your legs flat on the floor.

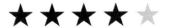

★ ★ ★ ★ ☆

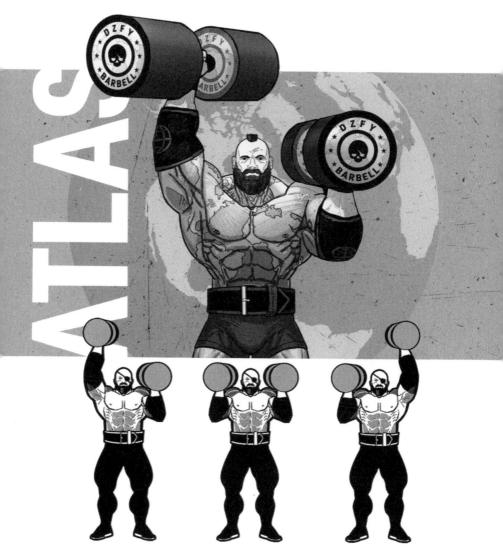

DUMBBELL ALTERNATING SHOULDER PRESSES
5 sets x 6 reps (2010) - rest 45s
(2s lower - 0 - 1s press - 0)

★ ★ ★ ★ ☆

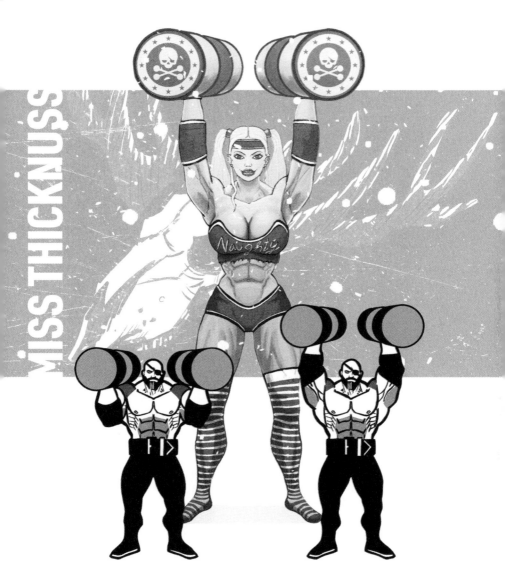

DUMBBELL STANDING SHOULDER PRESS
4 sets x 10 reps - rest 45s

TIP: Use full range of motion.
No half reps. Do not use your hips to cheat.

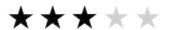

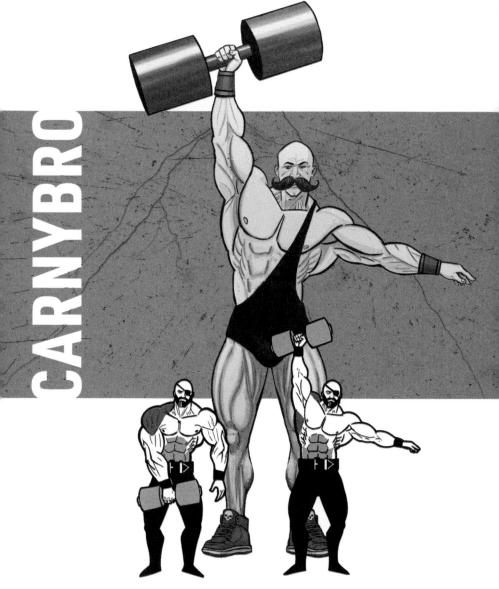

DUMBBELL SNATCH
(L/R; PYRAMID UP)
5 sets x 8 reps - rest 45s

TIP: To pyramid up, use 5 lbs/set.
Use your hips to snatch the dumbbell up.

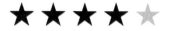
★ ★ ★ ★ ☆

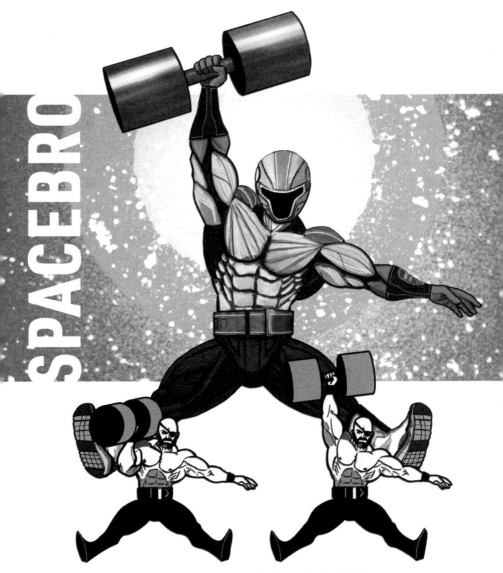

SPACEBRO

DUMBBELL FLOOR-SEATED SHOULDER PRESS (L/R)

4 sets x 8 reps (2010) - rest 60s

(2s lower - 0 - 1s press - 0)

TIP: Keep the other hand away from your body.

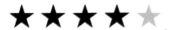

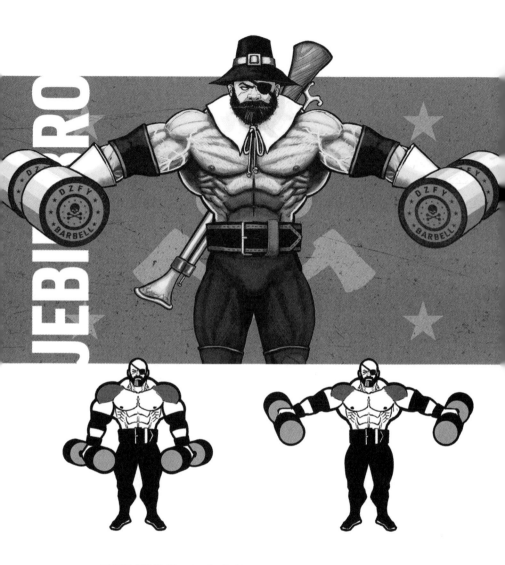

DUMBBELL SIDE LATERAL RAISES
5 sets x 5, 10 reps - rest 60s
(5 reps heavy, 10 reps 50% lighter.)

TIP: Raise to shoulder height.

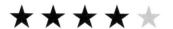

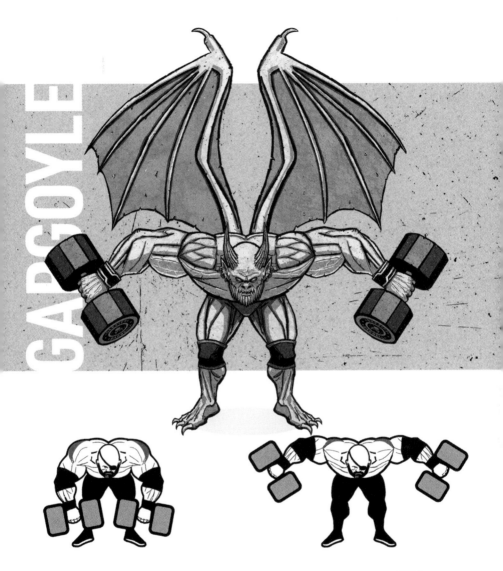

GARGOYLE

DUMBBELL BENT-OVER REVERSE FLYES
4 sets x 8 reps (2010) - rest 45s
(2s lower - 0 - 1s flye - 0)

TIP: Keep your back parallel to the floor.

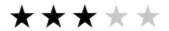

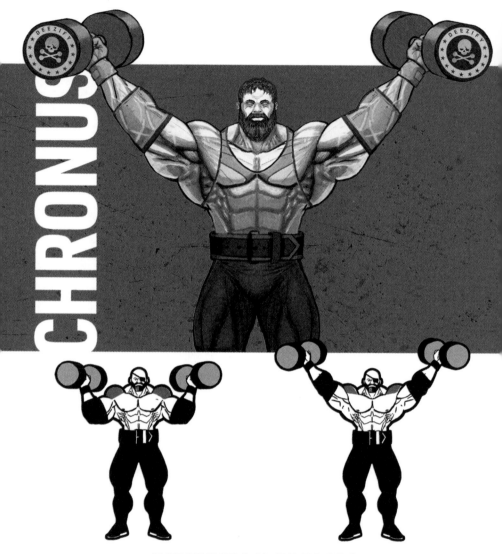

CHRONUS

DUMBBELL Y-PRESSES
4 sets x 8 reps (2010) - rest 45s
(2s lower - 0 - 1s press - 0)

TIP: Press out at a 45° angle.

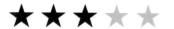

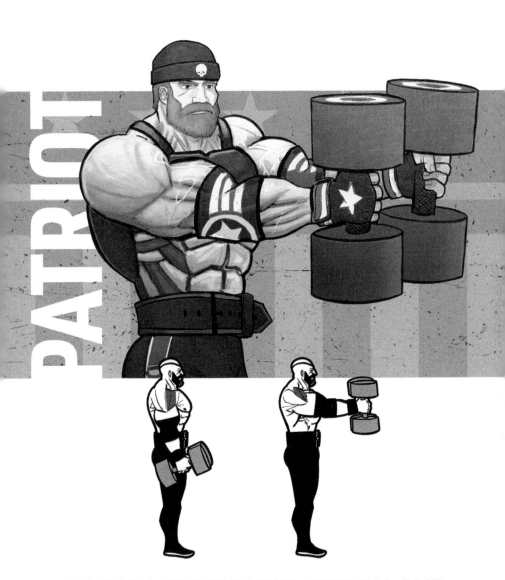

DUMBBELL FRONT RAISES—NEUTRAL GRIP

4 sets x 8 reps (2011) - rest 45s

(2s lower - 0 - 1s raise - 1s top hold)

TIP: Raise to shoulder height.

★★★☆☆

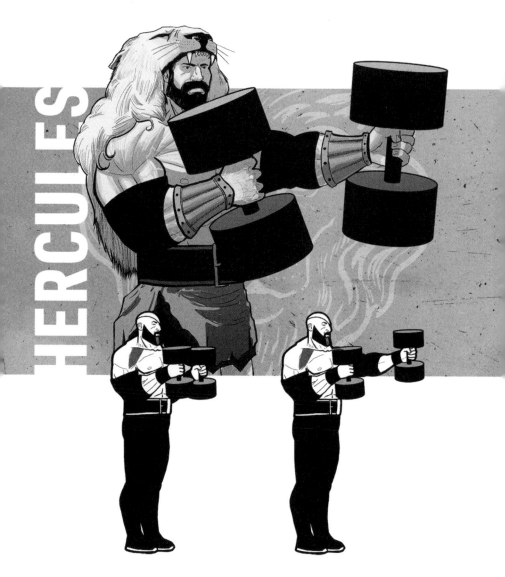

DUMBBELL SHOULDER PUNCHES
4 sets x 8 reps - rest 45s

TIP: Use a lighter weight.
VARIATION: Double punch.

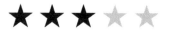

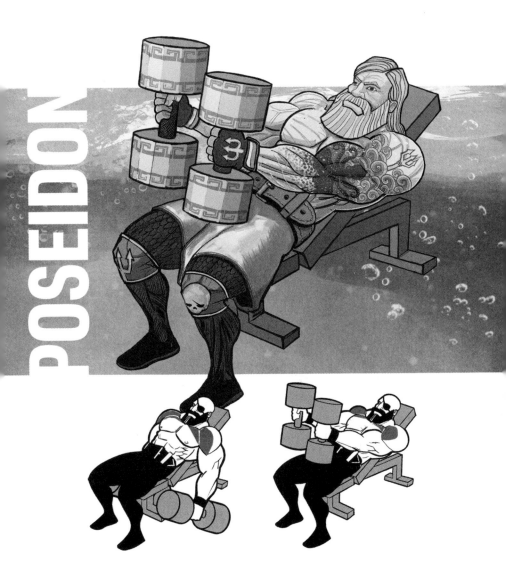

POSEIDON

DUMBBELL FRONT RAISES ON INCLINE BENCH

4 sets x 8 reps (2010) - rest 45s

(2s lower - 0 - 1s raise - 0)

TIP: The incline bench should be at a 30° to 45° angle.

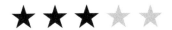

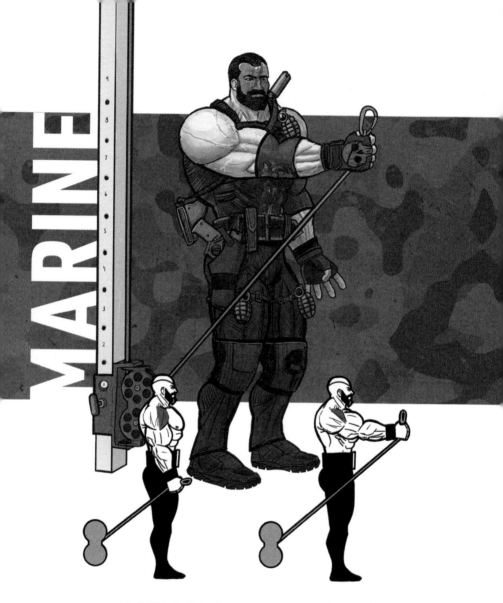

CABLE FRONT RAISES (L/R)
4 sets x 10 reps (2011) - rest 45s
(2s lower - 0 - 1s raise - 1s top pause)

TIP: Raise to shoulder height only.

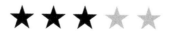

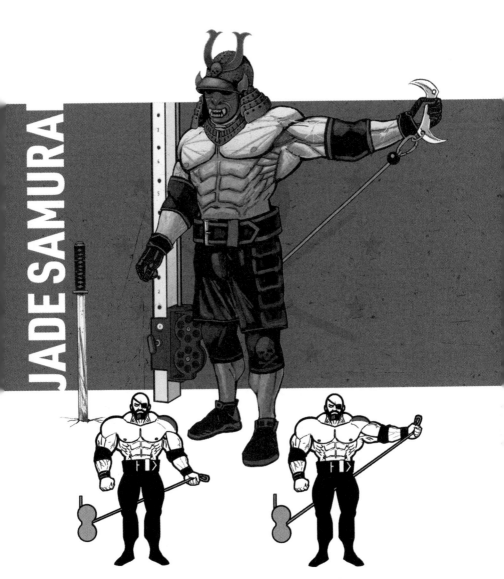

JADE SAMURAI

CABLE SIDE LATERAL RAISES (L/R)

4 sets x 10 reps (2011) - rest 45s

(2s lower - 0 - 1s raise - 1s top pause)

TIP: Raise to shoulder height only.

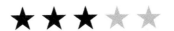

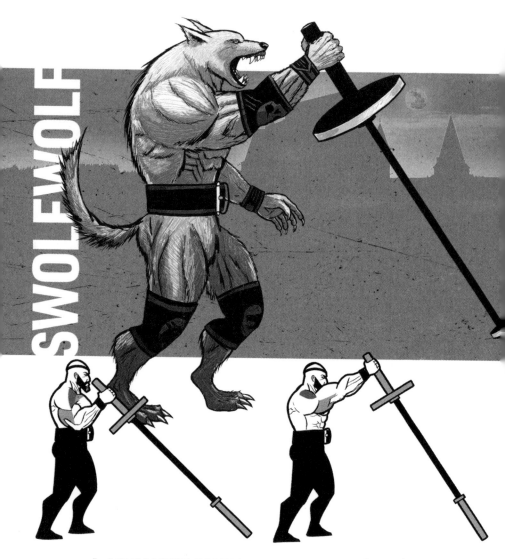

SWOLFWOLF

LANDMINE SHOULDER PRESS (L/R)
4 sets x 10 reps (2010) - rest 45s
(2s lower - 0 - 1s press - 0)

TIP: Can use barbell hack against the wall.

★ ★ ★ ☆ ☆

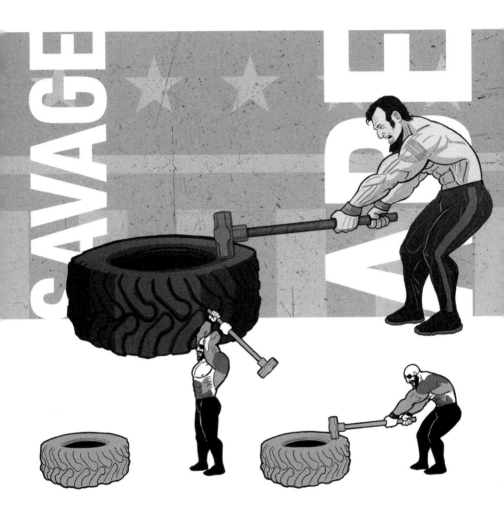

HAMMER SLAMS (LEFT, RIGHT, OVERHEAD)
4 sets x 10, 10, 10 reps - rest 60s
(10 left hand, 10 right hand, 10 overhead slams, rest.)

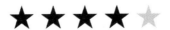

SHOULDER EXERCISES SUMMARY

BARBELL SHOULDER PRESS
3 sets x 8 reps - rest 60s

MOD
· Shoulder-Press Machine

SET
· **Strength:** 4 sets x 10 reps
· **Power:** 5 sets x 5 reps

BARBELL FLOOR-SEATED SHOULDER PRESS
4 sets x 8 reps - rest 60s

SET
· **Basic:** 4 sets x 10 reps with just the Olympic bar
· **Heavy:** 10, 8, 6, 6, 6 reps - rest 60s

DUMBBELL ALTERNATING SHOULDER PRESSES
5 sets x 6 reps (2010) - rest 45s
· (2s lower - 0 - 1s press - 0)

MOD
· Dumbbells or Kettlebells: Double presses or single-arm presses
· **Basic:** Single-arm shoulder-press machine presses

SET
· 4 sets x 8 reps - rest 60s

DUMBBELL STANDING SHOULDER PRESS
4 sets x 10 reps - rest 45s

MOD
· Kettlebells
· **Basic:** Shoulder-press machine presses

SET
· 4 sets x 8 reps - rest 60s

DUMBBELL SNATCH (L/R; PYRAMID UP)
5 sets x 8 reps - rest 45s

MOD
· Kettlebell Snatches

SET
· **Power:** 3 sets x 6 reps - rest 60s

DUMBBELL FLOOR-SEATED SHOULDER PRESS (L/R)
4 sets x 8 reps (2010) - rest 60s
· (2s lower - 0 - 1s press - 0)

MOD
· Kettlebell Floor-Seated Shoulder Press (L/R)
· Double-Dumbbell Floor-Seated Shoulder Press

SET
· 4 sets x 10-8 reps - rest 45s

DUMBBELL SIDE LATERAL RAISES
5 sets x 5,10 reps - rest 60s
· 5 reps heavy, 10 reps 50% lighter

SET
· 4 sets x 10 reps (2010) - rest 45s
· 4 sets x 8 reps - rest 45s

DUMBBELL BENT-OVER REVERSE FLYES
4 sets x 8 reps (2010) - rest 45s
· (2s lower - 0 - 1s flye - 0)

MOD
· **Machine Reverse Flyes:** Keep a little bend in the elbows.

SET
· 4 sets x 10-8 reps - rest 45s
· **Compound Set:** Dumbbell Shoulder Presses, Front Raises, or Side Lateral Raises

DUMBBELL Y-PRESSES

4 sets x 8 reps (2010) - rest 45s
· (2s lower - 0 - 1s press - 0)

MOD
· Change angle of press from Y
  to T for more challenge.

SET
· **Compound Set:** Side Lateral Raises
  - 3 sets x 8, 8 reps - rest 60s

DUMBBELL FRONT RAISES–NEUTRAL GRIP

4 sets x 8 reps (2011) - rest 45s
· (2s lower - 0 - 1s raise - 1s top hold)

MOD
· **Barbell Front Raises:** Hold the
  barbell in a palm-up grip.
· Cable Front Raises L/R

SET
· **Strength:** 4 sets x 10 reps - rest 45s
· **Compound Set:** Cable Side Lateral Raises/
  DB Front Raises -
  4 sets x 8, 8 reps - rest 60s

DUMBBELL SHOULDER PUNCHES

4 sets x 8 reps - rest 45s

MOD
· Use a lighter weight.
· Double punches or alternating punches

SET
· **Basic:** 4 sets x 10 reps - rest 45s

DUMBBELL FRONT RAISES ON INCLINE BENCH

4 sets x 8 reps (2010) - rest 45s
· (2s lower - 0 - 1s raise - 0)

MOD
· Use lighter dumbbells and adjust
  the incline for different angles.

CABLE FRONT RAISES (L/R)

4 sets x 10 reps (2011) - rest 45s
· (2s lower - 0 - 1s raise - 1s top pause)

MOD
· **Barbell Front Raises:** Hold the
  barbell in a palm-up grip.
· **Dumbbell Front Raises:** Double-
  arm or alternating raises

SET
· **Strength:** 4 sets x 10 reps - rest 45s
· **Compound Set:** Cable Side Lateral
  Raises - 4 sets x 8, 8 reps - rest 60s

CABLE SIDE LATERAL RAISES (L/R)

4 sets x 10 reps (2011) - rest 45s
· (2s lower - 0 - 1s raise - 1s top pause)

MOD
· **Dumbbell Side Raises:** Double-
  arm or alternating raises
· Machine Side Lateral Raises

SET
· **Strength:** 4 sets x 10 reps - rest 45s
· **Compound Set:** Cable Front Raises
  - 4 sets x 10, 10 reps - rest 60s

LANDMINE SHOULDER PRESS (L/R)

4 sets x 10 reps (2010) - rest 45s
· (2s lower - 0 - 1s press - 0)

SET
· **Power:** 3 sets x 8 reps - rest
  60s - explosive press
· **Hypertrophy:** 4 sets x 10 reps - rest 45s

HAMMER SLAMS (LEFT, RIGHT, OVERHEAD)

4 sets x 10, 10, 10 reps - rest 60s
· 10 left hand, 10 right hand,
  10 overhead slams, rest

SET
· 4 sets x 30s, 30s, 30s - rest 60s
  (time-based sets)

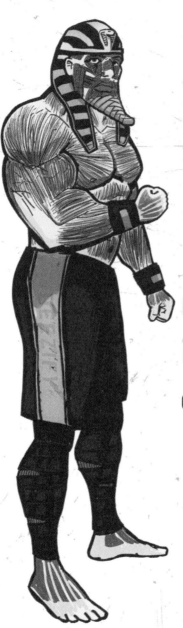

WORK
like a slave.
COMMAND
like a king.
CREATE
like a god.

Constantin Brancusi

ARMS

BICEPS EXERCISES

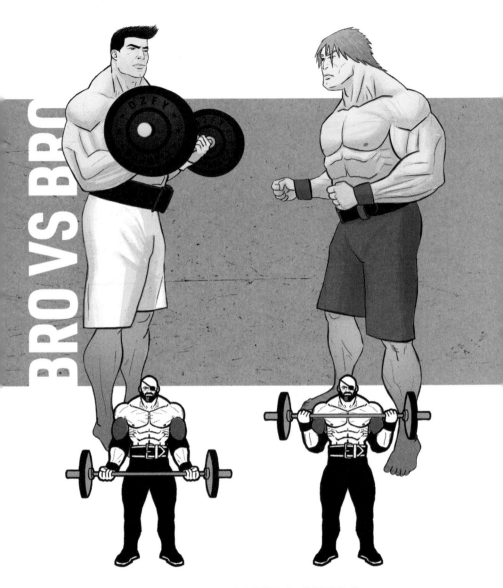

BARBELL BICEPS CURLS
3 sets x AMRAP - back and forth

TIP: No rest. Best of 3 wins.
For intensity, try 20+ reps.

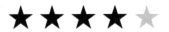

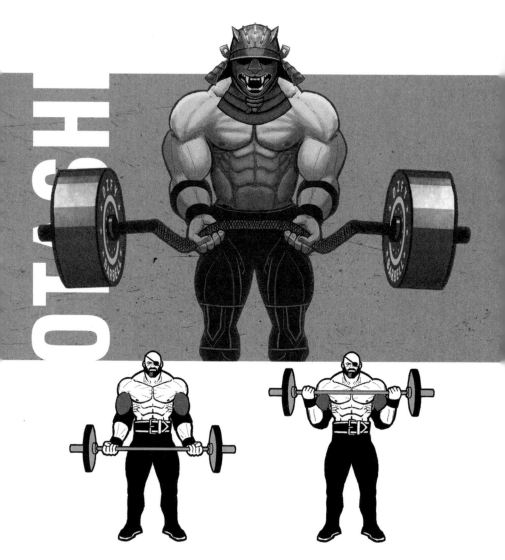

BARBELL BICEPS CURLS (PYRAMID UP)

6 sets x 10–4 reps - rest 45s

(Increase 10 lbs/set to 4 reps max.)

TIP: Keep your form strict. No body English.

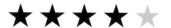

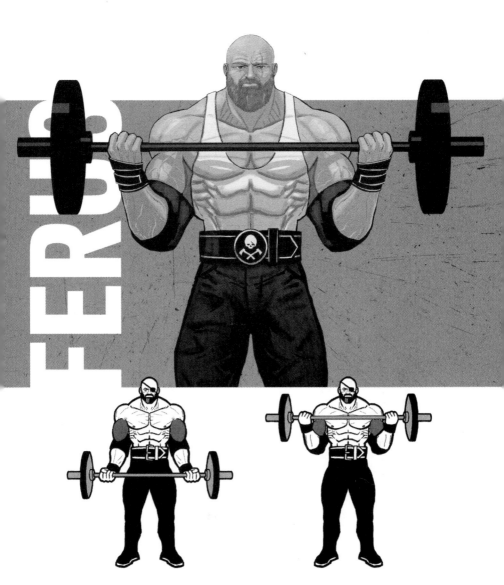

BARBELL BICEPS CURLS (STRIP SET)
4 sets x 10, 10, 10 reps - rest 60s
(Decrease 20% per drop (e.g.: 100, 80, 60 lbs).)

★ ★ ★ ★ ☆

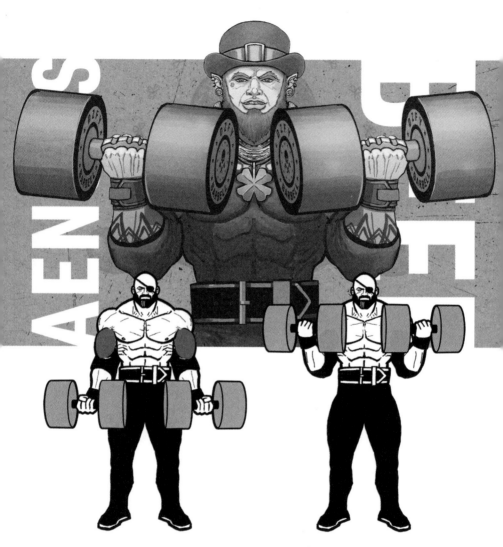

DUMBBELL BICEPS CURLS (RUN RACK UP)

6 sets x 10-4 reps - rest 20s

(Increase 5 lbs/set until 4 reps max.)

TIP: Keep your form strict. No body English.

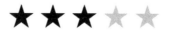

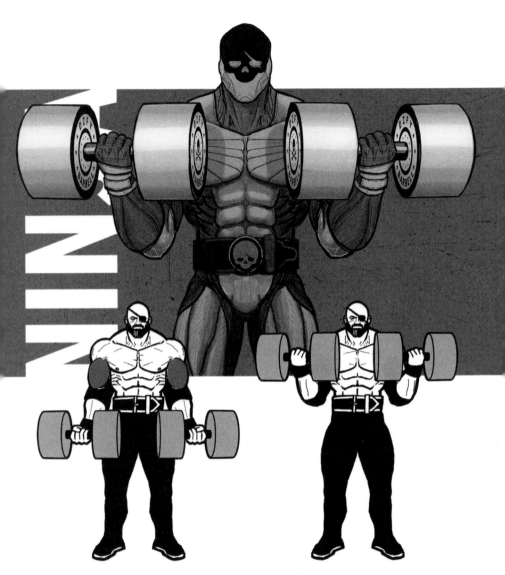

DUMBBELL BICEPS CURLS (UP AND DOWN)

6 sets x 6, 6, 6 reps - rest 60s

(On 1st, 3rd, 5th set, pyramid up 5 lbs/set.
On 2nd, 4th, 6th set, pyramid down 5 lbs/set.)

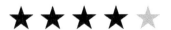

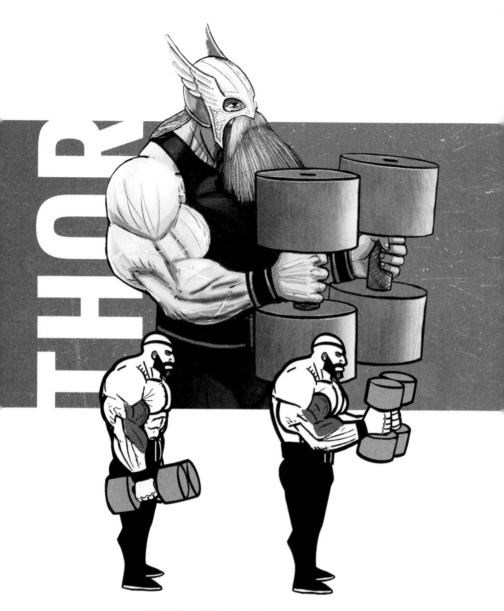

DUMBBELL HAMMER CURLS
Run rack up x 6 reps/set - rest 30s
(Run rack down x AMRAP/set - no rest.
Increase/decrease 5 lbs/set.)

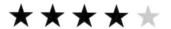

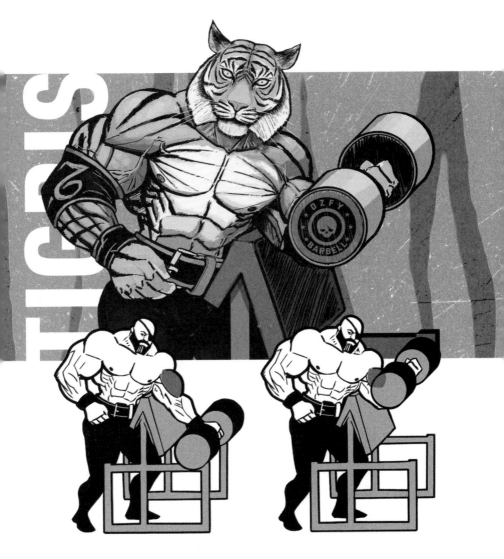

DUMBBELL PREACHER BICEPS CURLS (L/R)
4 sets x 6 reps (3010) - rest 45s
(3s lower - 0 - 1s curl - 0)

TIP: Build up with 2 or 3 warm-up sets,
then perform 4 sets of 6 reps.

★ ★ ★ ☆ ☆

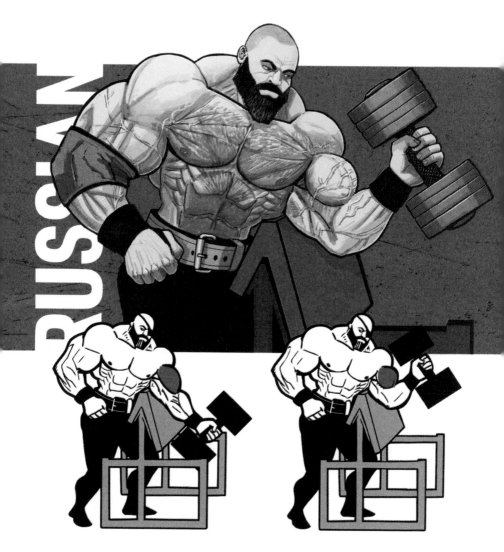

DUMBBELL PREACHER HAMMER CURLS (L/R)
4 sets x 8 reps (2010) - rest 45s
(2s lower - 0 - 1s curl - 0)

TIP: Keep tension on the biceps.

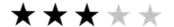

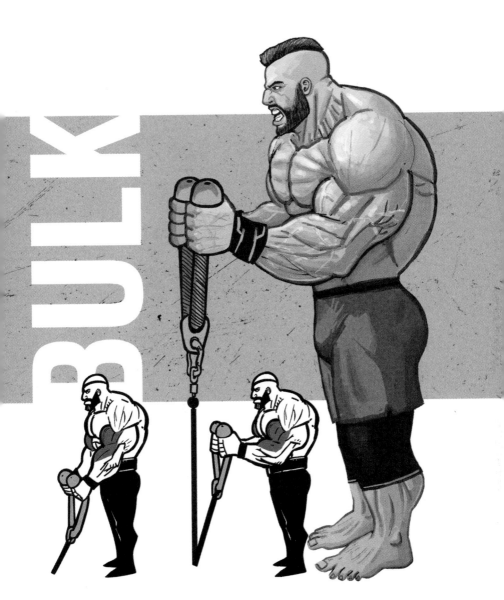

BULK

CABLE/ROPE HAMMER CURLS
5 sets x 10 reps (2012) - rest 60s
(2s lower - 0 - 1s curl - 2s top hold)

TIP: Contract and hold at the top of the curl.

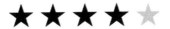

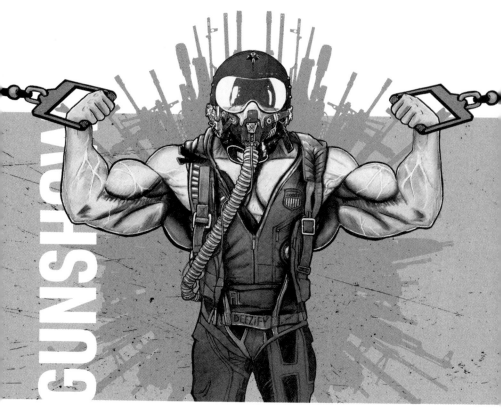

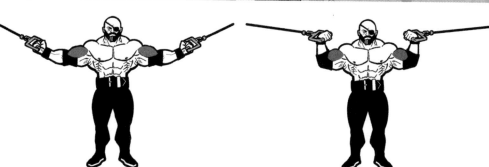

CABLE/HANDLE DOUBLE BICEPS CURLS
4 sets x 10 reps - rest 45s
(Increase 5 lbs/set to 4 work sets.)

TIP: Set the cable/handles at eye level.

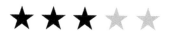

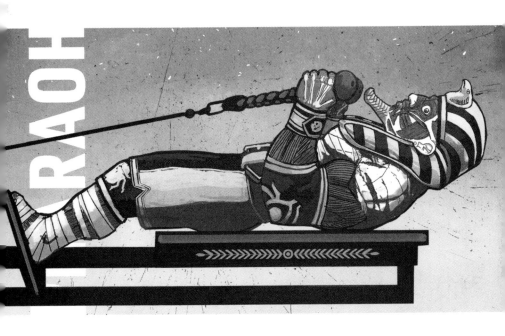

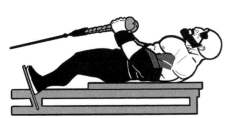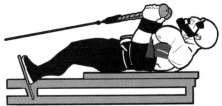

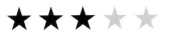

CABLE/ROPE LAYING HAMMER CURLS

4 sets x 8 reps (3010) - rest 30s

(3s lower - 0 - 1s curl - 0)

TIP: Keep your elbows tucked in.

★ ★ ★ ☆ ☆

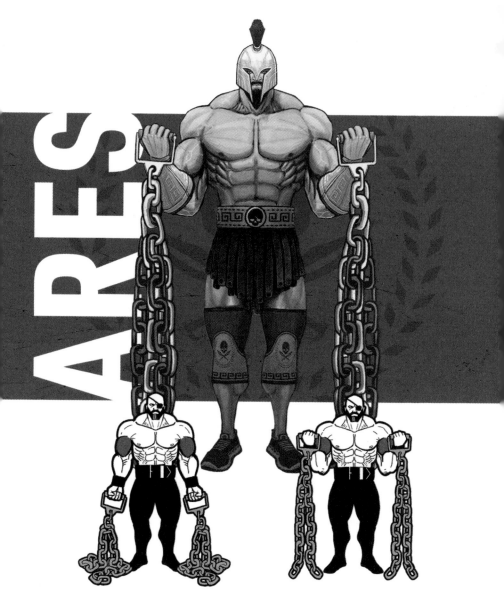

CHAIN BICEPS CURLS
4 sets x 10 reps - rest 45s

TIP: Adjust length for weight distribution.

★★★★☆

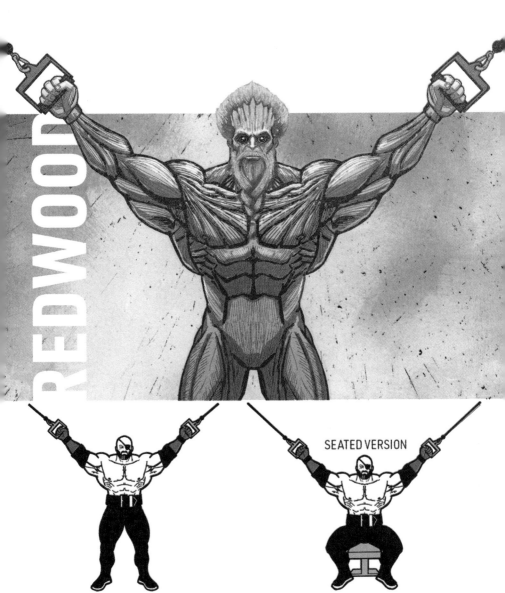

REDWOOD

SEATED VERSION

CABLE/ROPE HERCULES HOLD
5 sets x 20s hold - rest 60s

TIP: Hold heavy weight for iron grip.
Sit on bench if required.

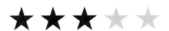

BICEPS EXERCISES SUMMARY

BARBELL BICEPS CURLS
3 sets x AMRAP - back and forth -
no rest - best of 3 wins
· I also call this back-and-forth partner
biceps curl "circuit penitentiary curls."
Two competing workout partners help
push each other. Everyone benefits
from some healthy competition.

MOD
· Can add a third friend; one person
passes the bar to another.

SET
· 3 sets x 20-30 reps - rest 30s
for single-person workout

BARBELL BICEPS CURLS
(PYRAMID UP)
6 sets x 10-4 reps - rest 45s
· A 10-lb increase per set is a good
increase per set for the buildup.

MOD
· Use EZ-Curl or straight bars,
changing it up for each workout.

SET
· Heavy, 4-6 reps; medium,
6-10 reps; light, 10+ reps

BARBELL BICEPS CURLS
(STRIP SET)
4 sets x 10, 10, 10 reps - rest 60s
· Strip sets can be performed more
easily with plates or cable pin stacks.
20% is usually a good drop. However,
sometimes a plate (or pin
drop) is more convenient, as
you don't want to rest between
the strip sets (drop set).

MOD
· **Cable/Bar Biceps Curls:** easier
to change weights.

SET
· **Beginner:** 3 sets x 10, 10, 10 reps

DUMBBELL BICEPS CURLS
(RUN RACK UP)
6 sets x 10-4 reps - rest 20s

MOD
· Double curls or alternating curls.
· **Seated curls on bench:** This eliminates
body English momentum cheating.

SET
· 6 reps/set (Run Rack Up) + 5 lbs/set
and AMRAP/set (Run Rack Down) -
10 lbs/set
· **Hypertrophy:** 4 sets x 8 reps (3010)
- rest 45s - 3s negatives

DUMBBELL BICEPS CURLS
(UP AND DOWN)
6 sets x 6, 6, 6 reps - rest 60s

MOD
· **Size:** 4 sets x 10, 10, 10 reps -
rest 60s - 5-lb differences.
· **Drop Set:** 4 sets 10, 10 reps - rest 60s.
· **Heavy:** 10 reps followed by 10 lighter reps.

DUMBBELL HAMMER CURLS
Run Rack Up x 6 reps/set - rest 30s

MOD
· Double Hammer Curls or
Alternating Hammer Curls
· **Seated hammer curls on the
bench:** This eliminates body
English momentum cheating.

SET
· **Size:** 4 sets x 8 reps (3010) -
rest 45s - 3s negatives

DUMBBELL PREACHER BICEPS CURLS (L/R)

4 sets x 6 reps (3010) - rest 45s
· (3s lower - 0 - 1s curl - 0)

MOD
· Double-Arm Biceps Curls
· Seated Preacher Curls or Machine Curls

SET
· 4 sets x 8 reps - rest 30s

DUMBBELL PREACHER HAMMER CURLS (L/R)

4 sets x 8 reps (2010) - rest 45s
· (2s lower - 0 - 1s curl - 0)

MOD
· Double-Arm Hammer Curls
· Seated Preacher Curls or Machine Hammer Curls

SET
· 4 sets x 8 reps - rest 30s

CABLE/ROPE HAMMER CURLS

5 sets x 10 reps (2012) - rest 60s
· (2s lower - 0 - 1s curl - 2s top hold)

SET
· 4 sets x 8 reps - rest 30s
· Superset with Rope Triceps Push-Downs

CABLE/HANDLE DOUBLE BICEPS CURLS

4 sets x 10 reps - rest 45s
· If you are tall, you may need to take a couple steps back to get a starting stretch in the biceps.

SET
· **Slower Tempo:** 4 sets x 8 reps (3010) - rest 45s
· **Pyramid Up:** 6 sets x 10–6 reps - rest 45s

CABLE/ROPE LAYING HAMMER CURLS

4 sets x 8 reps (3010) - rest 30s
· (3s lower - 0 - 1s curl - 0)
· Lie flat on your back to prevent any cheating.

MOD
· Use handles or bar for standard curls.

SET
· **Heavy:** 4 sets x 8–6 reps - rest 45s

CHAIN BICEPS CURLS

4 sets x 10 reps - rest 45s
· Chains involve a dynamic progressive overload method. As each link is lifted off the ground, it adds more weight to the lift. If all the links are off the ground, this adds a stability element because of the dangling and swinging nature of the chains, which add more difficulty as well.

MOD
· Stand on a box to get more height if you'd like to lift all the chain links.
· Can substitute with resistance bands for a progressive overload resistance.

SET
· 4 sets x 8 reps - rest 30s
· Add an isometric hold and contraction at the end of each rep for more stabilization work.

CABLE/ROPE HERCULES HOLD

5 sets x 20s hold - rest 60s

MOD
· Seated and kneeling stance; however, standing is recommended for heavy loads.

SET
· **Heavy:** 3 sets x hold for as long as possible - rest 60s

TRICEPS EXERCISES

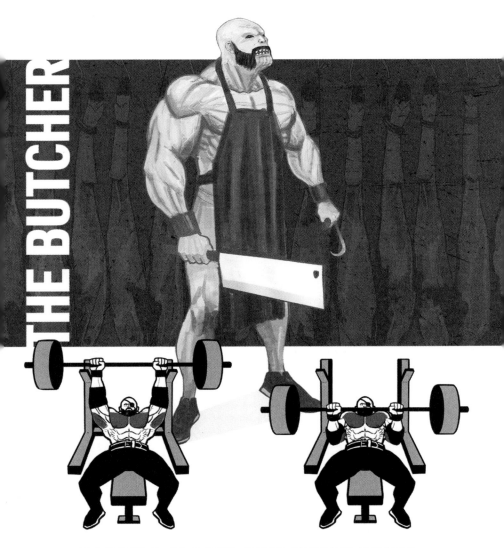

BARBELL CLOSER GRIP BENCH PRESS
10 sets x 10 reps (75% 1RM) - rest 45s

TIP: Only perform once every two weeks.
Keep your arms tucked in for triceps.

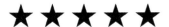

★ ★ ★ ★ ★

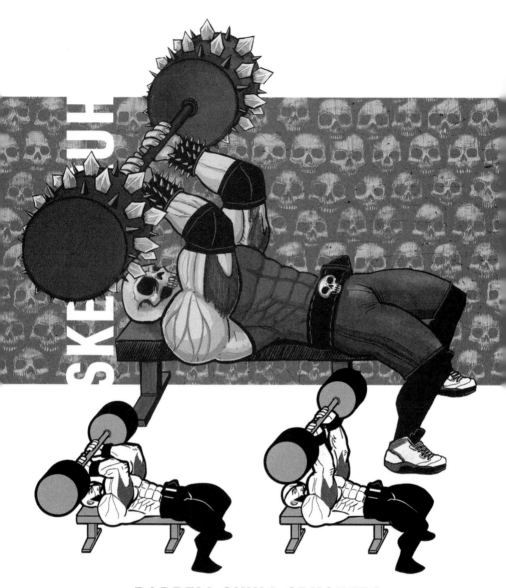

BARBELL SKULL CRUSHERS
4 sets x 10 reps (2010) - rest 45s
(2s lower - 0 - 1s lift - 0)

TIP: Lower toward the forehead.

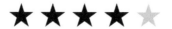

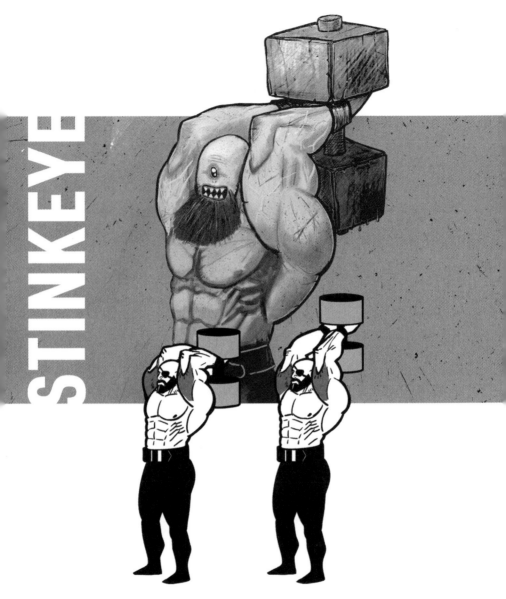

STINKEYE

DUMBBELL OVERHEAD TRICEPS PRESS
3 sets x 8 reps - rest 45s

TIP: To pyramid up, increase 10 lbs/set.
Perform 3 sets at 8 reps max.

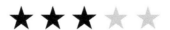

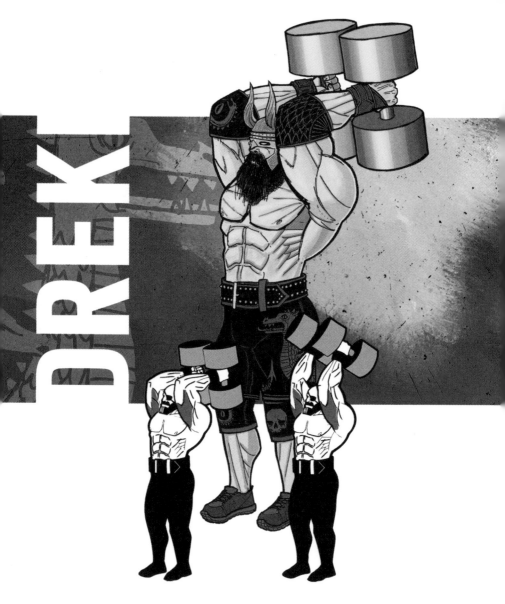

DUMBBELL OVERHEAD TRICEPS EXTENSIONS

4 sets x 10 reps (2010) - rest 45s

(2s lower - 0 - 1s lift - 0)

TIP: Keep your elbows pointed forward.

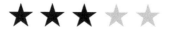

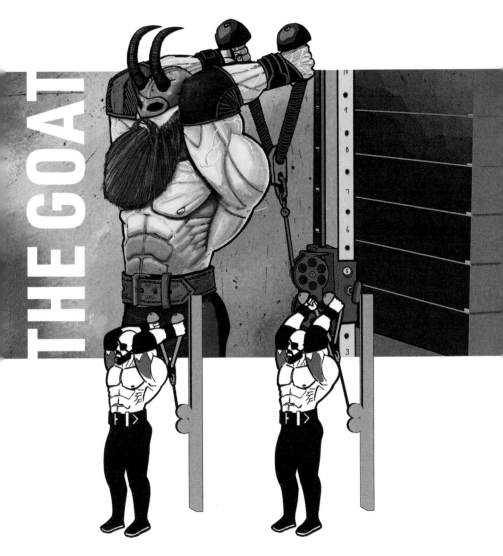

THE GOAT

CABLE/ROPE OVERHEAD TRICEPS EXTENSIONS
4 sets x 8 reps (2010) - rest 45s
(2s lower - 0 - 1s lift - 0)

TIP: Set up the rope attachment at hip level.

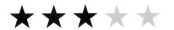

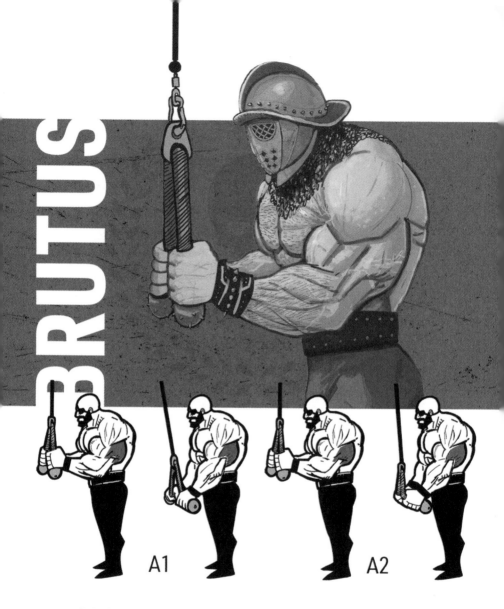

BRUTUS

A1

A2

A1 CABLE/ROPE TRI PUSH-DOWNS—OUT
A2 CABLE/ROPE TRI PUSH-DOWNS—DOWN
5 sets x 10, 10 reps - rest 60s

★ ★ ★ ☆ ☆

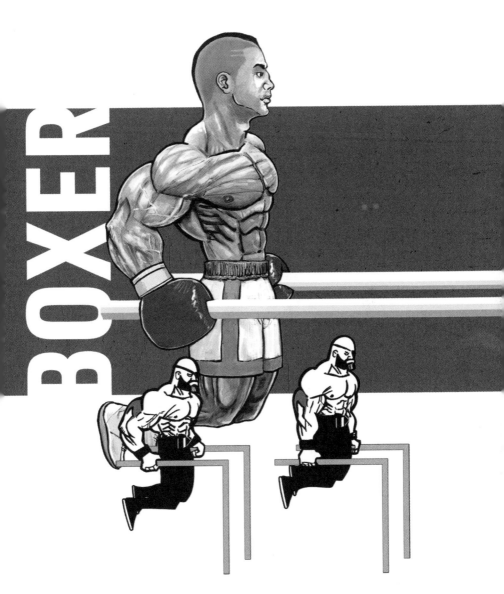

BOXER

TRICEPS DIPS—NEGATIVE ONLY
4 sets x 6 reps (8000) - rest 45s
(8s lower - 0 - 0 - 0)

TIP: Step up and then lower.
Keep your chest up and your feet back.

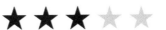

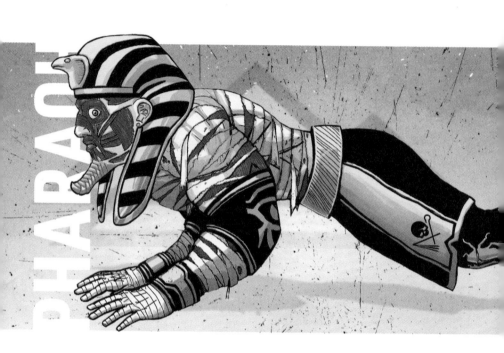

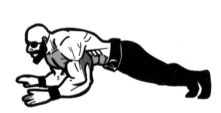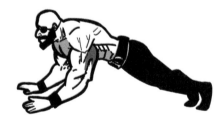

PHARAOH PUSH-UPS
4 sets x 10 reps (3010) - rest 45s
(3s lower - 0 - 1s push-up - 0)

TIP: Keep your elbows tucked in to your side.

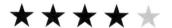

TRICEPS EXERCISES SUMMARY

BARBELL CLOSER GRIP BENCH PRESS
10 sets x 10 reps (75% 1RM) - rest 45s

MOD
· Move your hands closer
  together for triceps focus.

SET
· Power: 5 sets x 5 reps - rest 60s
· Strength: 4 sets x 10 reps

BARBELL SKULL CRUSHERS
4 sets x 10 reps (2010) - rest 45s
· (2s lower - 0 - 1s lift - 0)

SET
· Basic: 3 sets x 10 reps - rest 45s

DUMBBELL OVERHEAD TRICEPS PRESS
3 sets x 8 reps - rest 45s
· To pyramid up, increase 10 lbs/set.

MOD
· Basic: Seated overhead press;
  eliminates core from movement.
· Equipment: Can use EZ-Curl bar for variation.

SET
· 4 sets x 10 reps - rest 45s

DUMBBELL OVERHEAD TRICEPS EXTENSIONS
4 sets x 10 reps (2010) - rest 45s
· (2s lower - 0 - 1s lift - 0)

MOD
· Use the bench for a lying version. Lie down
  and extend your arms out from the bench.

SET
· 4 sets x 10 reps - rest 45s

CABLE/ROPE OVERHEAD TRICEPS EXTENSIONS
4 sets x 8 reps (2010) - rest 45s
· (2s lower - 0 - 1s lift - 0)
· Set up the rope attachment at hip level.
  The cable should be taut, stretching
  the triceps in the rest position.

MOD
· Can use a straight bar for variation.

SET
· 5 sets x 10-6 reps - rest 45s

A1 CABLE/ROPE TRI PUSH-DOWNS-OUT
A2 CABLE/ROPE TRI PUSH-DOWNS-DOWN
5 sets x 10, 10 reps - rest 60s

MOD
· Can perform these individually
  instead of as a compound set.
· Reverse order of exercises (e.g.: Push-
  Downs-Down; then Push-Downs-Out)

SET
· Hypertrophy: 4 sets x 8 reps (3010)
  - rest 60s - 3s negatives

TRICEPS DIPS-NEGATIVE ONLY
4 sets x 6 reps (8000) - rest 45s
· (8s lower - 0 - 0 - 0)
· Step up and lower.

MOD
· Basic: Assisted Dip Machine
· Equipment: Dip Machine

SET
· Basic: 4 sets x 10 reps - rest 60s
· Hard: 4 sets x AMRAP - rest 45s

PHARAOH PUSH-UPS
4 sets x 10 reps (3010) - rest 45s
· (3s lower - 0 - 1s push-up - 0)

MOD
· Basic: Support your upper body
  on a raised surface.
· Basic: Push-ups with your
  elbows tucked by your side.

SET
· Strength: 4 sets x AMRAP - rest 60s

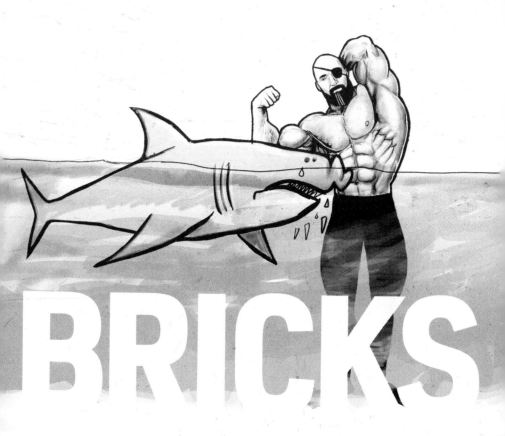

BRICKS

CORE

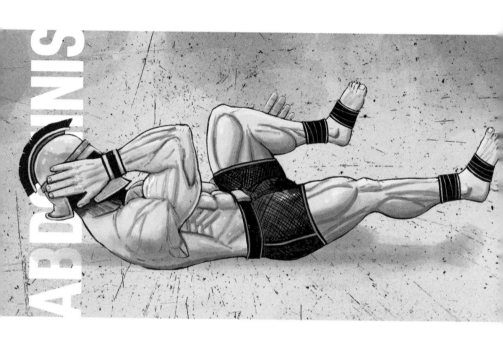

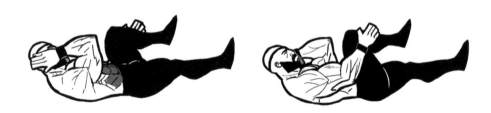

AB SPRINTERS
4 sets x 30s - rest 45s

TIP: Alternate your arms and feet quickly.
Extend your legs without touching the floor.

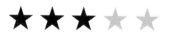

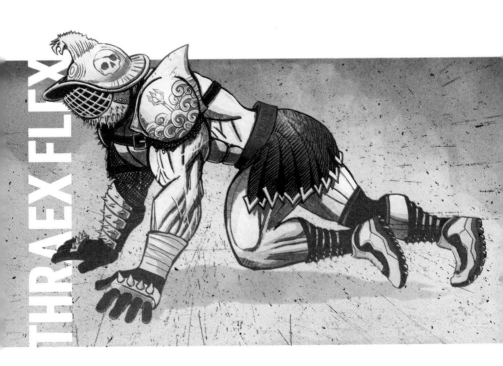

THRAEX FLEX

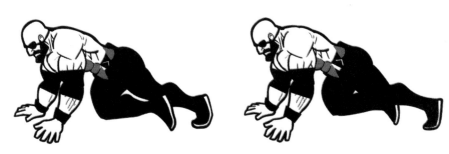

MOUNTAIN CLIMBERS
4 sets x 45s - rest 45s

TIP: Alternate your feet quickly,
and drive your knees forward.

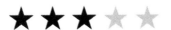

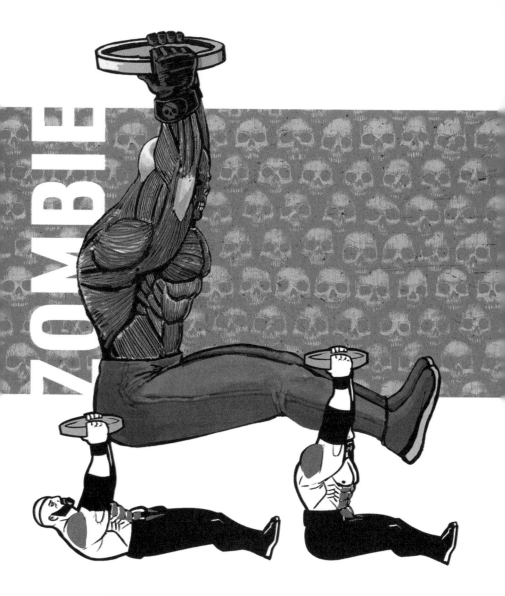

WEIGHT-PLATE COFFIN SIT-UPS
4 sets x 10 reps (3010) - rest 45s
(3s lower - 0 - 1s sit-up - 0)

TIP: Keep the plate high as though it's glued to the ceiling.

★ ★ ★ ☆ ☆

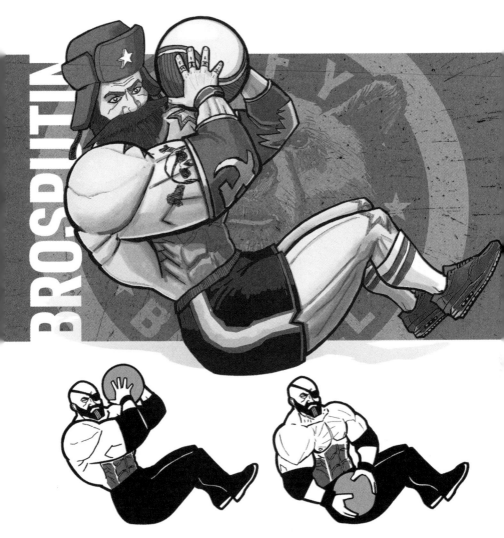

BROSPUTIN

MEDICINE BALL WOODCHOPPERS (L/R)
4 sets x 60s (30s/side) - rest 45s
(Left shoulder to right hip/right shoulder to left hip.)

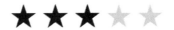

★ ★ ★ ☆ ☆

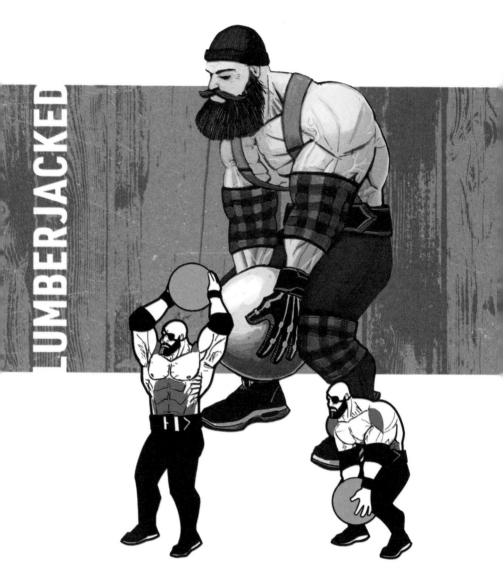

MEDICINE BALL WOODCHOPPERS
4 sets x 45s (or 20 reps) - rest 45s

TIP: Lift the medicine ball overhead (inhale),
and chop down with force (exhale).

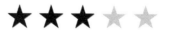

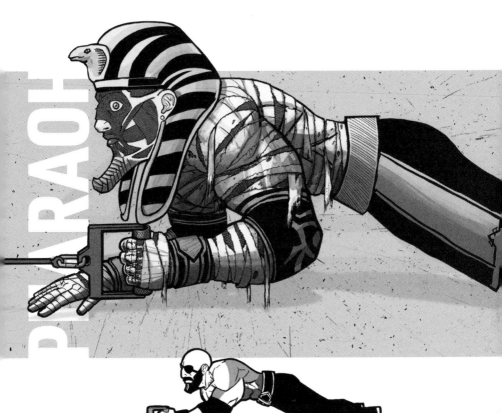

PHARAOH

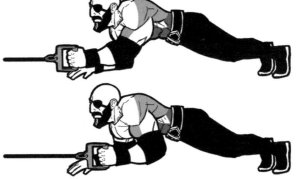

CABLE/HANDLE PLANK ROWS
4 sets x 8 reps (3011) - rest 45s
(3s lower - 0 - 1s row - 1s squeeze)

TIP: Can substitute with a resistance band.

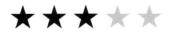

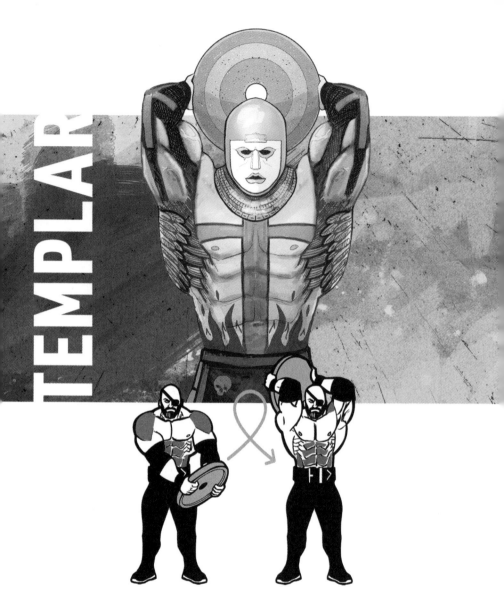

TEMPLAR

PLATE RIBBONS
4 sets x 10 reps - rest 45s

TIP: The ribbon motion goes from the hip to around the head. Do left to right and then right to left.

★ ★ ★ ☆ ☆

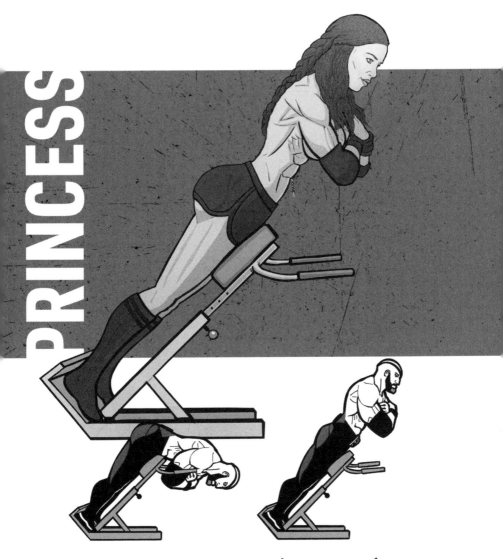

45° BACK RAISES (WARM UP)
5 sets x 20 reps - rest 30s
(100 total reps)

TIP: Use your bodyweight only.
This targets the lower back, glutes, and hams.

CORE EXERCISES SUMMARY

AB SPRINTERS
4 sets x 30s - rest 45s
- Your feet should never touch the ground as you alternate your legs and arms.

SET
- 4 sets x 20 reps total (1210) - rest 45s
  - pause for 2s with extended leg

MOUNTAIN CLIMBERS
4 sets x 45s - rest 45s

MOD
- **Beginner:** Place your hands on a raised platform for easier upper-body support.

SET
- **Beginner:** 3 sets x 30s - rest 30s
- **Endurance:** 3 sets x 20 reps - rest 45s

WEIGHT-PLATE COFFIN SIT-UPS
4 sets x 10 reps (3010) - rest 45s
- (3s lower - 0 - 1s sit-up - 0)
- Keep the plate glued high to the ceiling, with your arms always raised and bending at the hips.

MOD
- **Regression:** Perform the movement without any weight at first.

SET
- 4 sets x 15 reps

MEDICINE BALL WOODCHOPPERS (L/R)
4 sets x 60s (30s/side) - rest 45s

MOD
- **Russian twist:** Tap the ball on the floor adjacent to your hips.
- Can use small dumbbell, kettlebell, or weight plate.

SET
- 4 sets x 30 reps total - rest 45s

MEDICINE BALL WOODCHOPPERS
4 sets x 45s (or 20 reps) - rest 45s

MOD
- **Medicine Ball Slam:** Woodchopper movement, but slam medicine ball to floor with each rep.

CABLE/HANDLE PLANK ROWS
4 sets x 8 reps (3011) - rest 45s
- (3s lower - 0 - 1s row - 1s squeeze)

MOD
- Attach a resistance band on a post instead of using a cable machine.
- **Regression:** Open up your feet for a wider footprint.

SET
- 4 sets x 15 reps - rest 45s

PLATE RIBBONS
· 4 sets x 10 reps - rest 45s
· The ribbon motion starts from one hip, transversely lifts across the torso, circles the back of the head, and transversely lowers down to the opposite hip.

MOD
· Can use a kettlebell, medicine ball, or weight plate.

SET
· 4 sets x 12–16 reps total - rest 45s

45° BACK RAISES (WARM UP)
5 sets x 20 reps - rest 30s
· Tap the ground with your fingers for appropriate range of motion. Inhale as you lower, exhale as you lift yourself.

SET
· **Warm-Up:** 5 sets x 20 reps or 4 sets x 25 reps (bodyweight only)
· 4 sets x 10 reps - rest 60s (weighted work sets)

ADDITIONAL NOTES:
· Many compound lifts work your core. Stop avoiding hard lifts and flocking to ab machines. A week on the machines makes you weak.
· Try to do as many exercises standing up or as many unilateral (one-sided) exercises as you can to engage your core throughout the exercise.
· Core exercises are great exercises to superset with bigger exercises or add to a circuit if you are tight on time.

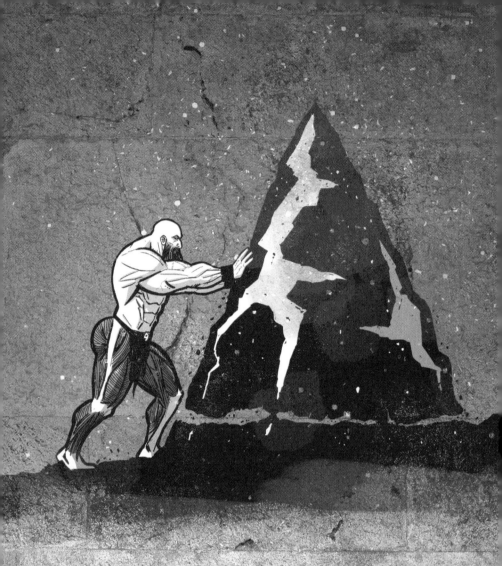

CRONUS WAS THE MOST
POWERFUL OF ALL TITANS.
BIG GLUTES MOVE
BIG MOUNTAINS.
NEVER SKIP LEG DAY.

LEGS

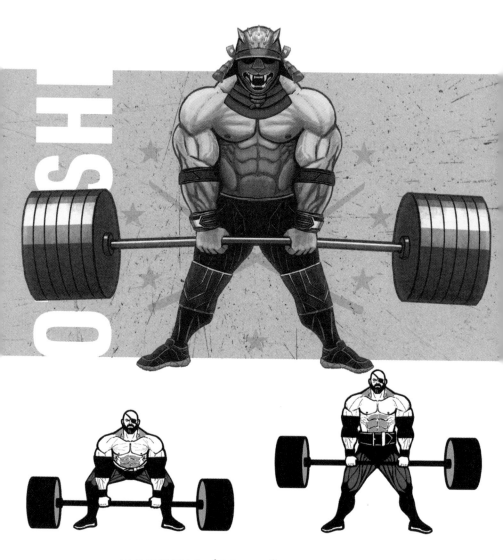

BARBELL (SUMO) DEADLIFTS
5, 5, 3, 3, 1 reps - rest 90s

TIP: Build up using 25-lb and 45-lb plates only.
Use sumo or conventional stance.

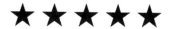

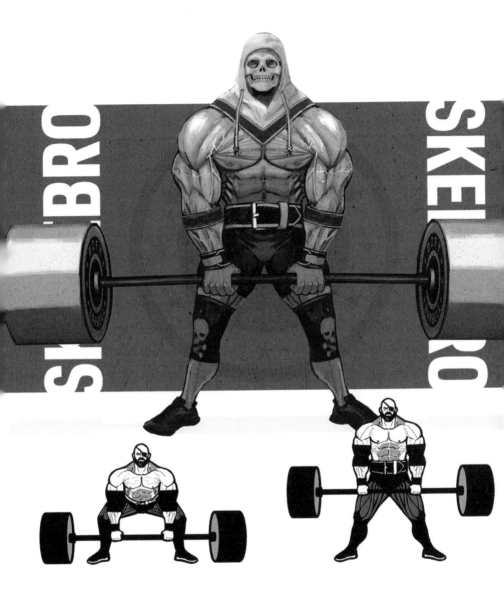

BARBELL (SUMO) DEADLIFTS
5, 3, 1, 1, 1 reps - rest 180s
(50%, 70%, 80%, 90%, 100% of 1RM)

TIP: Use sumo or conventional stance.

★ ★ ★ ★ ★

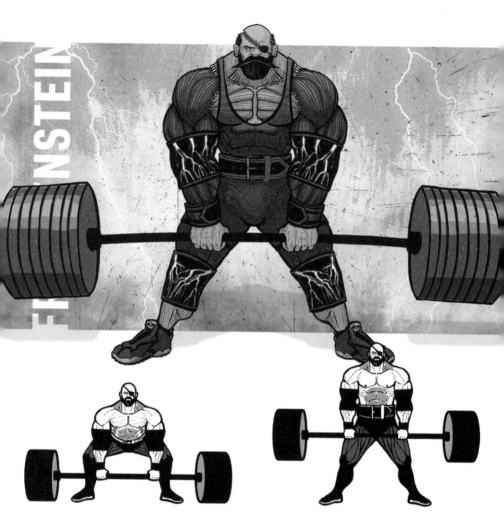

A. BARBELL (SUMO) DEADLIFTS
3 sets x 6 reps (75% 1RM) - rest 60s

B. BARBELL DEADLIFTS—SINGLES
3 sets x 1 rep (90% 1RM) - rest 120s

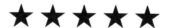

★ ★ ★ ★ ★

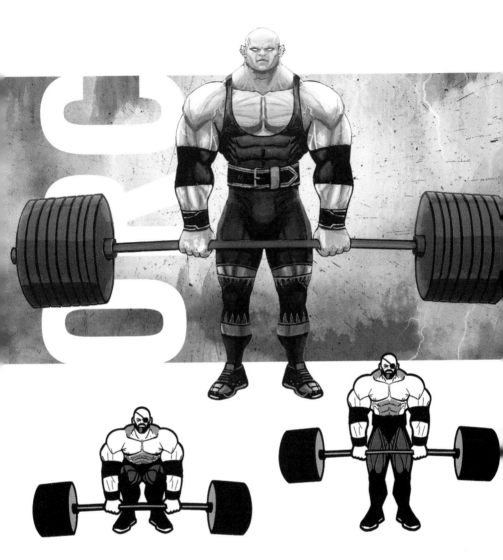

BARBELL (CONVENTIONAL) DEADLIFTS

1 set x AMRAP (85% 1RM) - rest 120s
4 sets x 6 reps (90% 1RM) - rest 120s
TIP: AMRAP = as many reps as possible

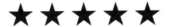

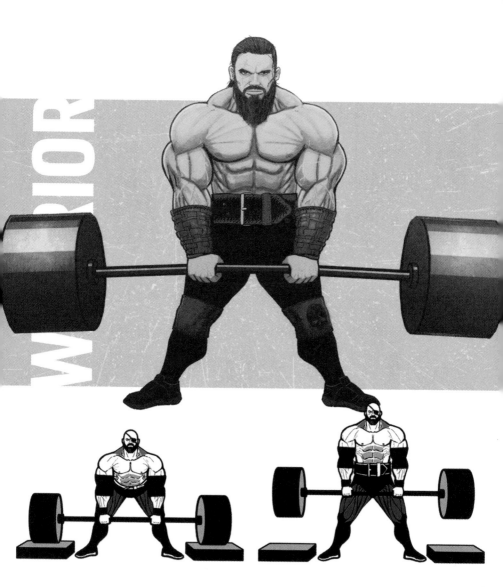

BARBELL RACK PULLS (SUMO)
3 sets x 3 reps - rest 90s

TIP: Set up blocks/pins at the deadlift sticking
point. Use your 1 rep max for deadlifts.

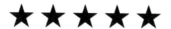

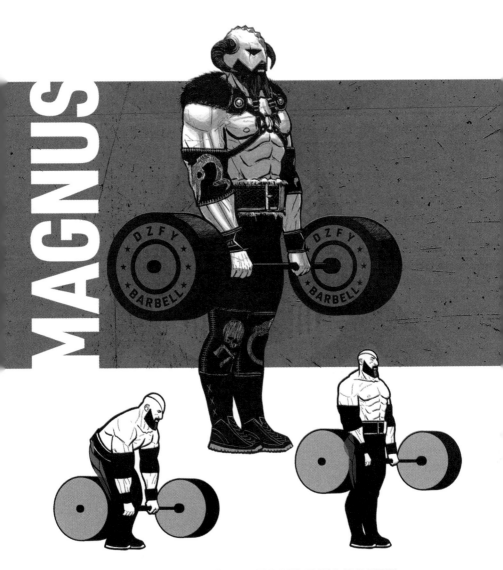

BARBELL ROMANIAN DEADLIFT
4 sets x 5 reps (30X0) - rest 90s
(3s lower - 0 - explosive lift - 0)

TIP: Stop 2 inches above the ground when lowering the barbell.

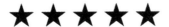

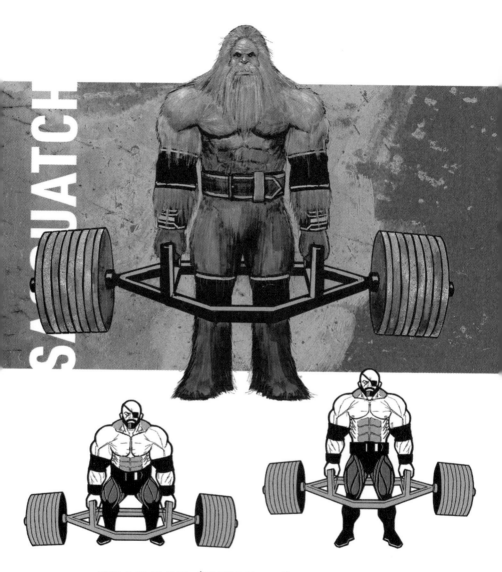

TRAP BAR (HEX BAR) DEADLIFTS
5 sets x 5 reps - rest 90s

TIP: Warm up and build up to 5 reps max.
Use raised handles to target your quads.

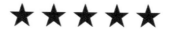

★ ★ ★ ★ ★

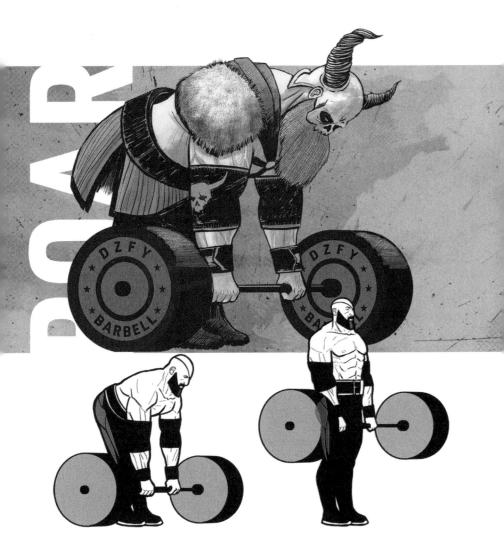

BARBELL STIFF-LEG DEADLIFTS
4 sets x 3 reps - rest 90s

TIP: Keep your back straight through the lift,
and build up appropriately.

★ ★ ★ ★ ★

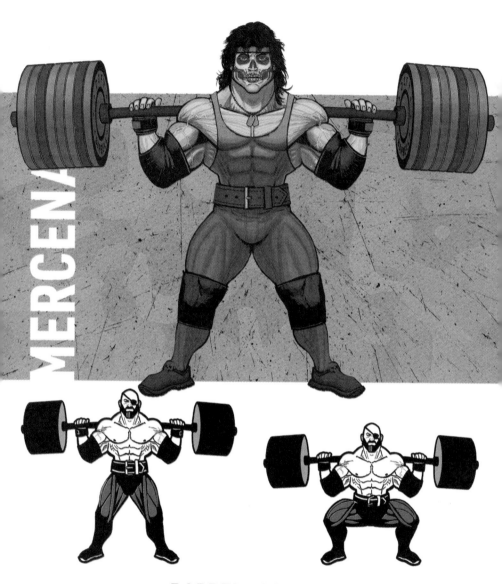

BARBELL SQUATS

5, 5, 5, 3, 3, 3 reps - rest 60s

TIP: Build up to 3 working sets of 3 reps.
Squat down so your thighs are parallel with the floor.

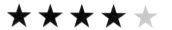

★ ★ ★ ★ ☆

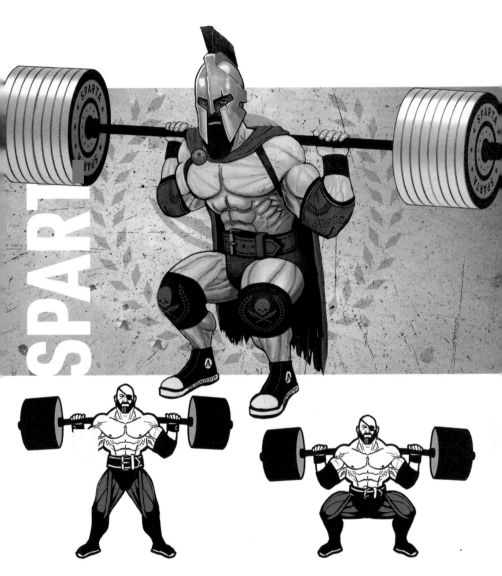

BARBELL SQUATS
4 sets x 6 reps - rest 60s

TIP: Use approximately 70–80% of 1 rep max.
Warm up and build up appropriately.

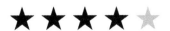

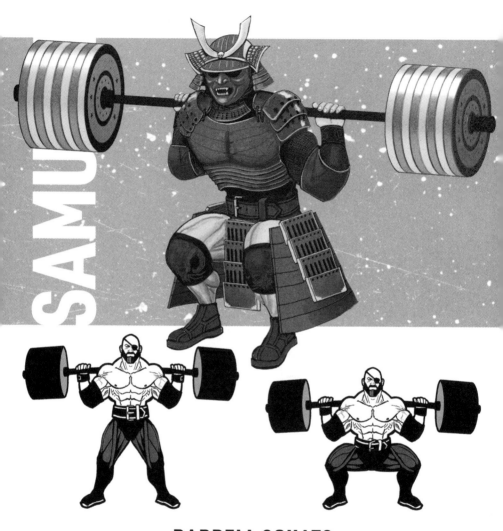

SAMU

BARBELL SQUATS
10 sets x 10 reps - rest 60s

TIP: Use approximately 70–80% of 1 rep max.
Perform only once every 2 weeks.

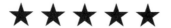

★ ★ ★ ★ ★

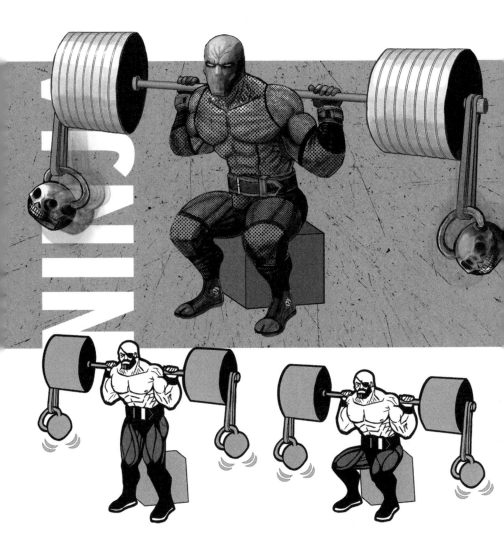

BARBELL BOX SQUATS WITH SUSPENDED WEIGHT
4 sets x 5 reps (3111) - rest 90s
(3s lower - 1s box pause - 1s squat - 1s pause at top)

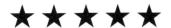

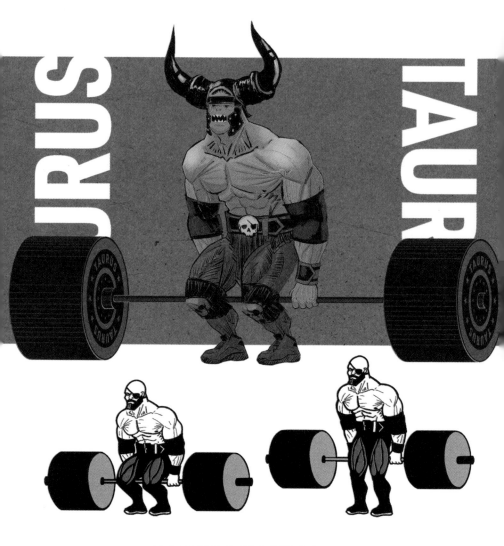

BARBELL HACK SQUAT
4 sets x 8 reps - rest 60s

TIP: The barbell and your hands should be behind your thighs.
Similar to deadlift with dead stop.

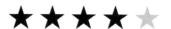

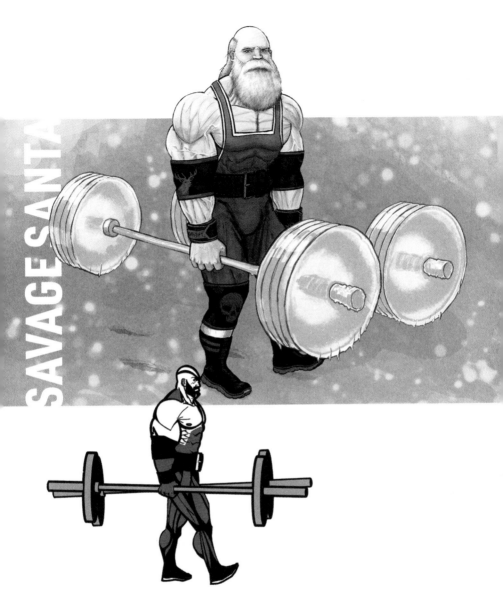

DOUBLE BARBELL FARMER'S WALK
4 sets x 60ft walk - rest 120s

TIP: Load both bars evenly, and attach clips. If the barbell tips and makes contact with the ground, put both barbells down. Reset, lift, and continue.

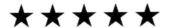

★ ★ ★ ★ ★

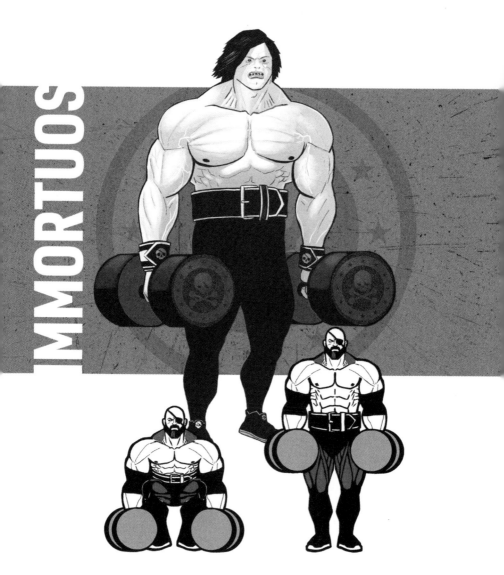

DUMBBELL SUITCASE DEADLIFTS
5 sets x 10 reps - rest 120s

TIP: Tap the ground with each rep.
Lift the dumbbells from the side.

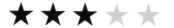

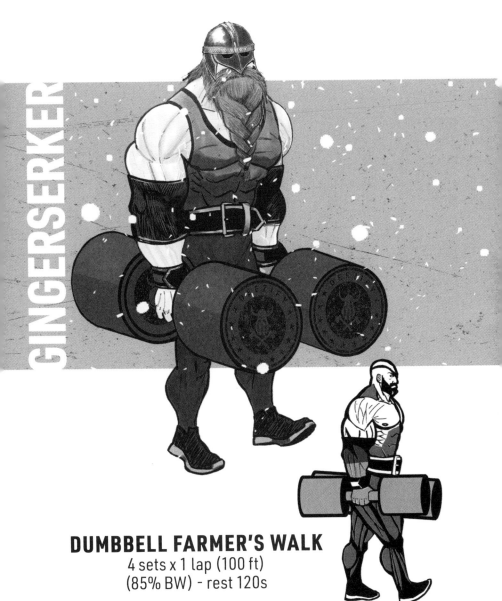

GINGERSERKER

DUMBBELL FARMER'S WALK
4 sets x 1 lap (100 ft)
(85% BW) - rest 120s

TIP: Use 85% of bodyweight (BW).
E.g.: if your bodyweight is 240 lbs, use
200 lbs total (2 x 100-lb DBs).

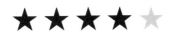

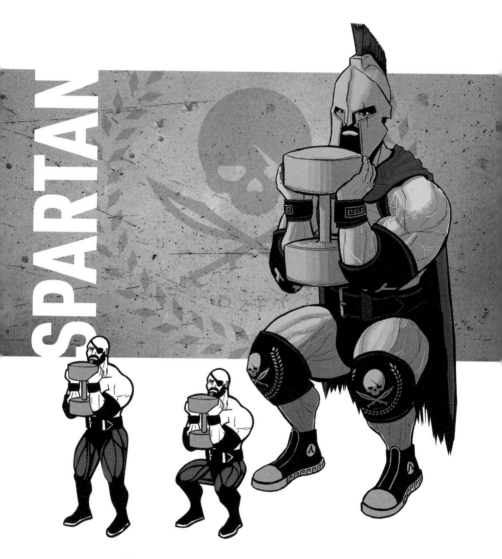

SPARTAN

DUMBBELL GOBLET SQUATS
5 sets x 20 reps - rest 60s

TIP: Can substitute with kettlebells.
Adjust your feet to squat more deeply.

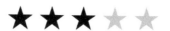

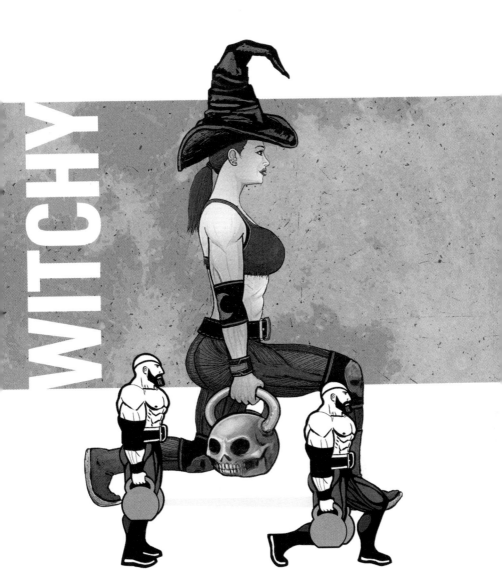

WITCHY

KETTLEBELL WALKING LUNGES
4 sets x distance (20 steps) - rest 60s

TIP: Target your glutes with a long step.
Target your quads with a short step.

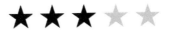

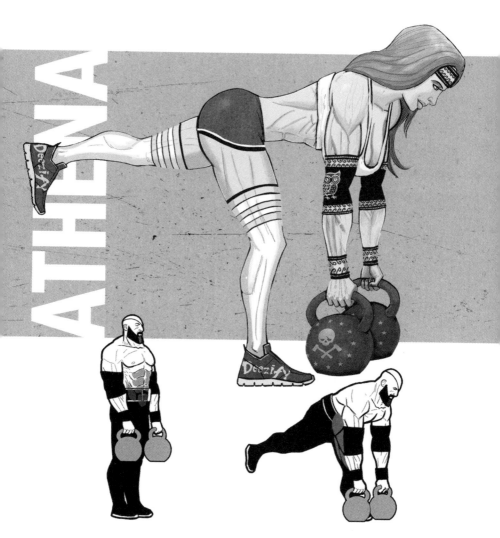

KETTLEBELL SINGLE LEG STIFF DEADLIFTS (L/R)

4 sets x 8 reps (3011) - rest 60s

(3s lower - 0 - 1s lift - 1s top pause)

TIP: Tap the ground with the kettlebells.

★ ★ ★ ☆ ☆

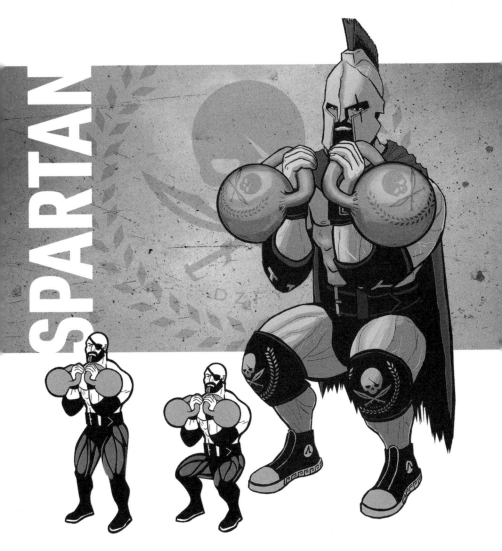

KETTLEBELL SQUATS
5 sets x 20 reps - rest 60s
(Men: Use 50 lbs+; women: use 35 lbs+.)

TIP: Keep the kettlebells in rack position.

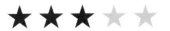

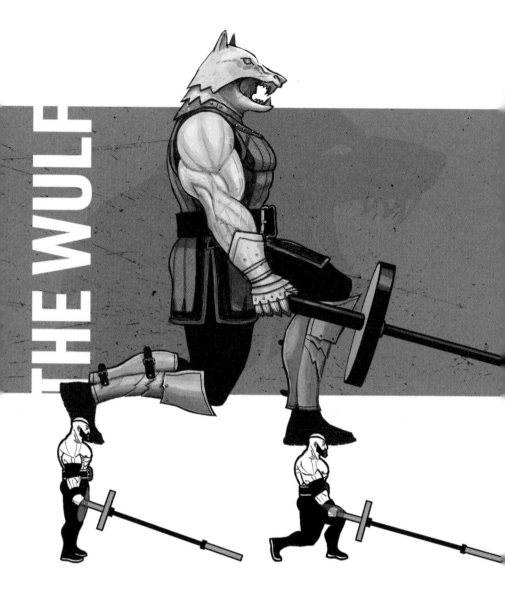

LANDMINE REVERSE LUNGES (L/R)

4 sets x 8 reps (3010) - rest 60s

(3s lower - 0 - 1s lift - 0)

TIP: The leg closest to the bar steps back.

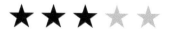

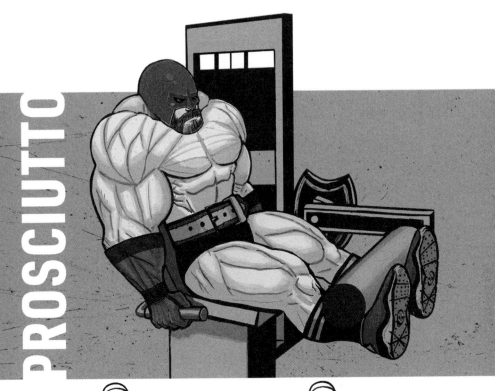

PROSCIUTTO

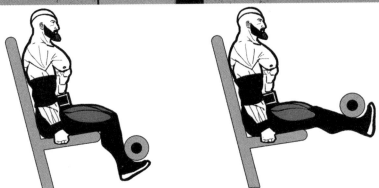

MACHINE LEG EXTENSIONS
4 sets x 10 reps (3010) - rest 45s
(3s lower - 0 - 1s lift - 0)

TIP: Keep the movement strict. No leg swinging.

★ ★ ★ ☆ ☆

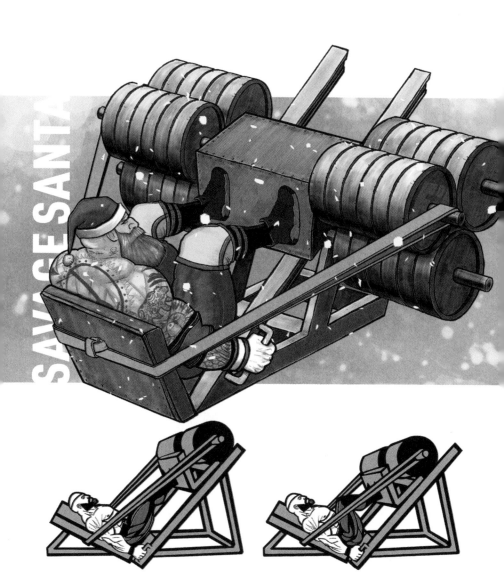

MACHINE LEG PRESS WITH BANDS
4 sets x 10 reps - rest 60s

TIP: Build up with 1 plate/set and then 4 work sets.

VARIATION: Regular leg press, no bands.

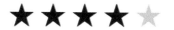

★ ★ ★ ★ ☆

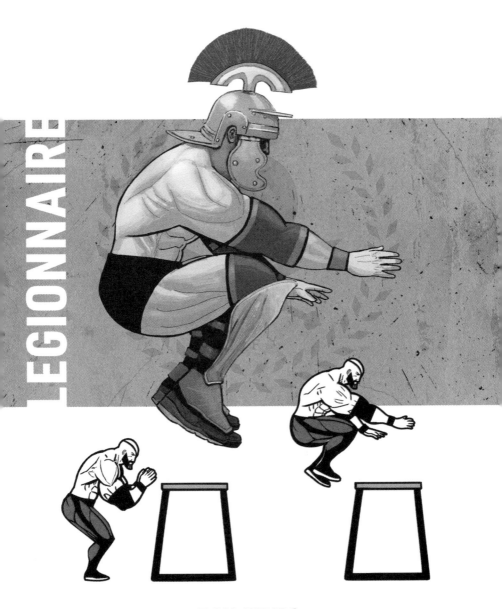

LEGIONNAIRE

BOX JUMPS
6 sets x 1–3 reps - rest 60s

TIP: Build up confidently and safely.
Step down if possible.

★ ★ ★ ★ ☆

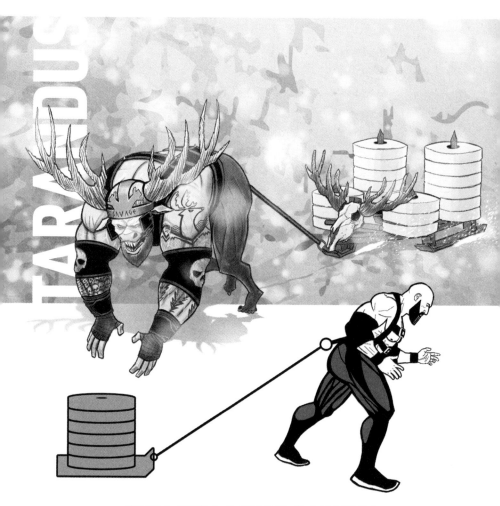

SLED PULLS WITH HARNESS
4 sets x 1 lap - rest 90s

TIP: Use approximately 70–80% of 1 rep max.
1 lap = 30–40 yards (100 ft)

★ ★ ★ ★ ☆

LEGS EXERCISES SUMMARY

BARBELL (SUMO) DEADLIFTS
5, 5, 3, 3, 1 reps - rest 90s - build up using 25-lb and 45-lb plates only.

BARBELL (SUMO) DEADLIFTS
5, 3, 1, 1, 1 reps - rest 180s - 50%, 70%, 80%, 90%, 100% of 1RM
· A Sumo Deadlift (as opposed to a Conventional Deadlift) is the deadlift lifting method but with a wider foot placement. The name originates from the sumo wrestler wide foot-stance pose. Never pull with your arms; they act like cables. Because of the wider stance, there is less stress on the lower back, especially for taller lifters. Practice both Sumo and Conventional Deadlifts in your workout routines.

MOD
· Conventional Barbell Deadlifts

SET
· **Power:** 5 sets x 5 reps - rest 180s
· **Power:** 3 sets x 3 reps - rest 180s
· **Strength:** 5 sets x 8 reps - rest 60s
· **Work:** 4 sets x 10 reps - rest 60s
· **Speed:** 8 sets x 3–2 reps - rest 60s

A BARBELL (SUMO) DEADLIFTS
3 sets x 6 reps (75% 1RM) - rest 60s

B BARBELL DEADLIFTS–SINGLES
3 sets x 1 rep (90% 1RM) - rest 120s

MOD
· Conventional Barbell Deadlifts

SET
· Pyramid Up to 1RM, then Drop Set Down 5, 5, 3, 1, 1, 3, 5, 5 reps

BARBELL (CONVENTIONAL) DEADLIFTS
1 set x AMRAP (85% 1RM) - rest 120s
· 4 sets x 6 reps (90% 1RM) - rest 120s
· AMRAP = as many reps as possible
· Conventional Deadlifts are deadlifts in which the feet are situated approximately shoulder-width apart. When pulling, the arms are always situated outside the thighs. It tends to be more of a quad- and lower-back-dominant pull, depending on one's height.

MOD
· Deficit Deadlifts on plate or block
· **Pause Deadlifts:** Pause for 1s mid shin.

BARBELL RACK PULLS (SUMO)
3 sets x 3 reps - rest 90s

MOD
· Rack Pulls on Raised Blocks
· Barbell Rack Pulls with Wide Snatch Grip

SET
· **Power:** 5, 5, 5, 3, 1, 1, 5 reps - rest 90s
· **Strength:** 4 sets x 8 reps - rest 60s

BARBELL ROMANIAN DEADLIFT
4 sets x 5 reps (30X0) - rest 90s
· (3s lower - 0 - explosive lift - 0)

MOD
· Barbell Romanian Deadlifts with wide snatch grip

TRAP BAR (HEX BAR) DEADLIFTS

5 sets x 5 reps - rest 90s
· Trap Bars (or Hex Bars) usually have 2 sets of handles. The higher handle raises the starting pull several inches higher. This starting height, similar to a rack pull, makes the lift easier since it alleviates lower-back stresses and the work path is reduced.

MOD
· Rack Pulls if trap bar is not available.
· Trap bars may have 2 sets of handles. The lower handle mimics regular deadlift height.

SET
· **Power:** 5, 5, 3, 3, 1 reps - rest 120s

BARBELL STIFF-LEG DEADLIFTS

4 sets x 3 reps - rest 90s

MOD
· **Deficit Stiff-Leg Deadlifts:** Stand on a 2-inch plate.

SET
· **Strength:** 4 sets x 8 reps - rest 60s

BARBELL SQUATS

5, 5, 5, 3, 3, 3 reps - rest 60s

BARBELL SQUATS

4 sets x 6 reps - rest 60s - approximately 70–80% of 1RM

BARBELL SQUATS

10 sets x 10 reps - rest 60s - approximately 70–80% of 1RM

MOD
· Can change your foot positions.

SET
· **Power:** 5 sets x 5 reps - rest 180s
· **Power:** 3 sets x 3 reps - rest 180s
· **Strength:** 5 sets x 8 reps - rest 60s
· **Endurance:** 4 sets x 10 reps - rest 60s
· **Speed:** 8 sets x 3–2 reps - rest 60s

BARBELL BOX SQUATS WITH SUSPENDED WEIGHT

4 sets x 5 reps (3111) - rest 90s
· (3s lower - 1s box pause - 1s squat - 1s pause at top)

MOD
· Squat to box with bottom pause, touch and go, or dead stop.

SET
· **Heavy:** 3 sets x 6 reps - rest 60s
· **Power:** 3 sets x 3 reps - rest 120s

BARBELL HACK SQUAT

4 sets x 8 reps - rest 60s
· Barbell Hack Squats are like deadlifts, as they are started from the ground in a dead stop. The bar is set up behind the feet, and the hands grasp the bar from behind. The placement of the bar targets the quadriceps more. Not everyone has the flexibility to get in the lifting position and perform this type of hack squat.

MOD
· Machine Hack Squats

DOUBLE BARBELL FARMER'S WALK

4 sets x 60-ft walk - rest 120s
· This Farmer's Walk is probably one of the most difficult exercises to perform. It tests your grip strength, your balance, your legs, your back—but, most importantly, your patience. The bars will tip and may touch and drag on the ground. If you lose your grip or a bar tips to the floor, put both bars down and reset. Lift and continue. Be sure to have plenty of walking area.

MOD
· Use Farmer's Walk bars or dumbbells.

DUMBBELL SUITCASE DEADLIFTS

5 sets x 10 reps - rest 120s

MOD
· Trap Bar Deadlifts or Kettlebell Suitcase Deadlifts

SET
· 5 sets x 20 reps - rest 60s

DUMBBELL FARMER'S WALK
4 sets x 1 lap (100 ft)
(85% BW) - rest 120s

MOD
· Dumbbell Farmer's Walks
  with Weighted Vest
· Kettlebell Farmer's Walk with Racked
  Kettlebells (held above waist)

DUMBBELL GOBLET SQUATS
5 sets x 20 reps - rest 60s

MOD
· Kettlebell Goblet Squats
· 2 Kettlebell Squats

SET
· **Strength:** 5 sets x 10 reps (3010) - rest 60s

KETTLEBELL WALKING LUNGES
4 sets x distance (20 steps) - rest 60s

MOD
· **Glutes:** long step; **quads:** short step
· Hold KB or DB by the side or in rack
  position, with the barbell across the
  back; use chains or a weighted vest.
· KB or DB Standing Alternating Lunges
  (no walking - lunge forward, step back)

SET
· 4 sets x 16 steps (3010) - rest 60s

KETTLEBELL SINGLE-LEG
STIFF DEADLIFTS (L/R)
4 sets x 8 reps (3011) - rest 60s
· (3s lower - 0 - 1s lift - 1s top pause)

MOD
· Single-leg double dumbbells, single-leg
  single KB or DB, single-leg barbell

SET
· 4 sets x 10 reps - rest 60s
· **Heavy:** 3 sets x 6 reps

KETTLEBELL SQUATS
5 sets x 20 reps - rest 60s

MOD
· **Recommended weight:** Men should use
  50 lbs+; women should use 35lbs+.
· Kettlebell Goblet Squats
· 2 Kettlebell Squats

SET
· **Strength:** 5 sets x 10 reps (3010) - rest 60s

LANDMINE REVERSE LUNGES (L/R)
4 sets x 8 reps (3010) - rest 60s
· (3s lower - 0 - 1s lift - 0)

MOD
· **Basic:** Use the bar only.

SET
· 4 sets x 10 reps - rest 60s

MACHINE LEG EXTENSIONS
4 sets x 10 reps (3010) - rest 45s
· (3s lower - 0 - 1s lift - 0)

MOD
· Single-Leg Machine Leg Extensions

SET
· 5 sets x 20 reps - rest 60s

MACHINE LEG PRESS WITH BANDS
4 sets x 10 reps - rest 60s

MOD
· Standard Leg Press (without bands)

SET
· **Hypertrophy:** 10 sets x 10 reps
· **Pyramid Up:** 10 reps/set; increase
  1 plate/set to 5 reps max

BOX JUMPS
6 sets x 1-3 reps - rest 60s

SET
· **Warm Up:** 3 sets x 5 reps - rest
  45s (with smaller box height)

SLED PULLS WITH HARNESS
4 sets x 1 lap (70-80% of 1RM) - rest 90s
· 1 lap = 30-40 yards

MOD
· Prowler/Sled Push if a
  harness isn't available

SET
· **Strength:** Pyramid Up 1 lap/set
  + add 1 plate/set - rest 90s
· **Work Capacity:** 10 laps with
  BW on sled - no rest

TO LIFT OR NOT TO LIFT THAT IS THE QUESTION

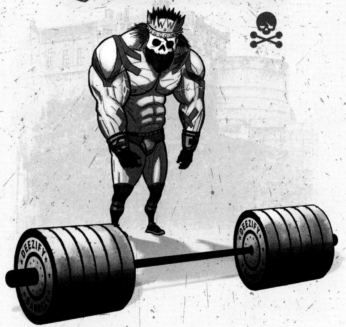

HELLS TO THEE YEA

WORKOUTS OF THE DAY (WODs)

CHEST GOD SACRIFICE

★ ★ ★ ★ ★

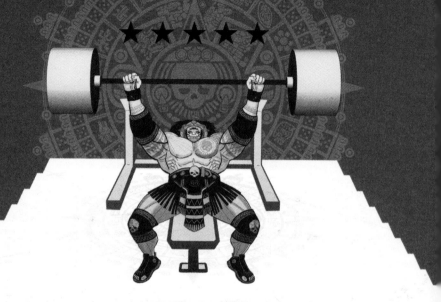

A. BARBELL BENCH PRESS
3 sets x 8 reps - rest 60s
Use your 10-rep max

B. BARBELL BENCH PRESS–EXTENDED SETS
3 sets x 8, 4, 2 reps - rest 60s
8 reps, rest 15s - 4 reps, rest 15s - 2 reps

C1. DUMBBELL INCLINE CHEST FLYES AT 30°
C2. DUMBBELL INCLINE CHEST PRESS AT 30°
3 sets x 8 reps - rest 60s

D1. DUMBBELL INCLINE CHEST FLYES AT 15°
D2. DUMBBELL INCLINE CHEST PRESS AT 15°
3 sets x 8 reps (2010) - rest 60s
(2s lower - 0 - 1s flye/press - 0)

E1. DUMBBELL CHEST FLYES AT 0°
E2. DUMBBELL CHEST PRESS AT 0°
3 sets x 8 reps (3010) - rest 60s
(3s lower - 0 - 1s flye/press - 0)

CHEST GOD SACRIFICE

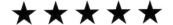

★ ★ ★ ★ ★

A: BARBELL BENCH PRESS

1. Lie back on the bench and grasp the bar with a grip that's a bit wider than shoulder-width apart.
2. With the bar grasped, ensure that your feet are on the floor and your upper back and head are in contact with the bench.
3. Retract your shoulder blades, and firmly brace your back against the bench.
4. When dismounting the bar, ensure that your eyes are positioned beneath the bar and that you extend your arms out.
5. Bend your arms and lower the barbell to your lower chest.
6. Lift the barbell up by extending your arms.
7. Repeat.
8. Rerack the barbell on the bench.

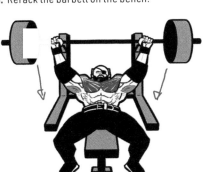

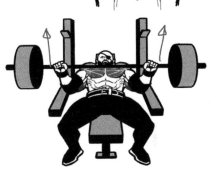

WARNING: Always have a spotter when attempting personal records or failure reps.

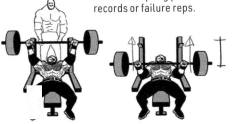

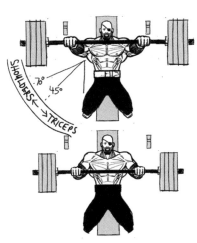

The angle of your arm to your torso will determine whether the press is more shoulder- (greater than 45°) or triceps-dominant (less than 45°).

Depending on your style of benching, this angle can range from 45° to 70°, while a closer grip bench press can range from 0° to 30°.

CHEST GOD SACRIFICE

★ ★ ★ ★ ★

C1, D1, AND E1: DB (INCLINE) CHEST FLYES 30°, 15°, 0°

1. Lie back on the bench with the dumbbells on your chest.
2. Extend your arms, lifting the dumbbells over your shoulders.
3. With a slight elbow bend, lower your arms in an arching motion so that they become parallel to the floor.
4. Lift by pulling your arms together and contracting your chest.
5. Repeat.

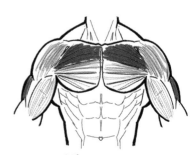

30° Bench Angle

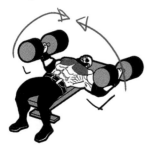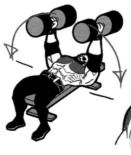

Bend your elbows while lowering. Straight-arm flyes may cause elbow hyperextension and rotator-cuff issues.

15° Bench Angle

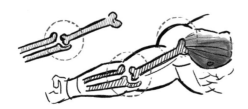

Bottom of Flye with Slight Elbow Bend and Tension

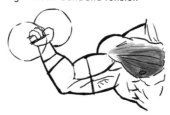

0° Flat Bench

CHEST GOD SACRIFICE

★ ★ ★ ★ ★

C2, D2, AND E2: DB INCLINE CHEST PRESS 30°, 15°, 0°

1. Lie back on the bench with the dumbbells on your chest.
2. Extend your arms, lifting the dumbbells over your shoulders.
3. Lower by bending your elbows down to your chest.
4. Lift by extending your arms and contracting your chest muscles.
5. Repeat.

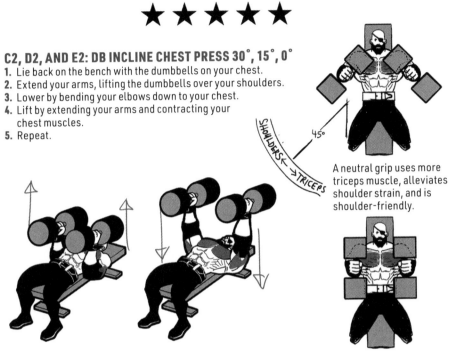

A neutral grip uses more triceps muscle, alleviates shoulder strain, and is shoulder-friendly.

Adjust the bench to your target muscles; anything above 45° will be shoulder-dominant and become a shoulder press.

TIP: Don't cheat and turn your shoulder presses into chest presses.

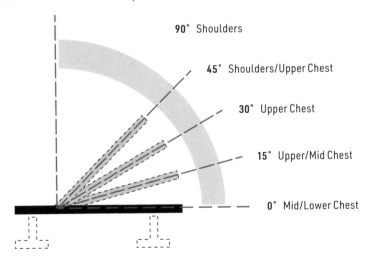

90° Shoulders

45° Shoulders/Upper Chest

30° Upper Chest

15° Upper/Mid Chest

0° Mid/Lower Chest

BACK ATTACK

★ ★ ★ ★ ★

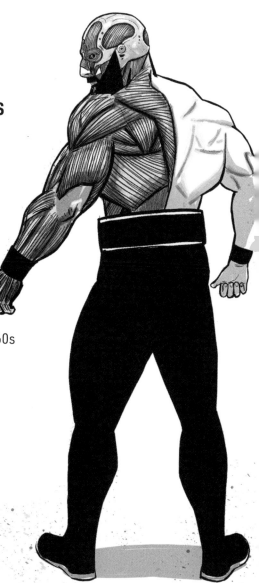

A. BARBELL PENDLAY ROWS
10, 10, 5, 5, 3, 3, 3, 3 reps - rest 90s
Keep your back parallel with the ground.

B. BARBELL 45° BACK RAISES
10, 10, 5, 5, 3, 3, 3, 3 reps - rest 90s
The reps start on the ground.

C1. CABLE/ROPE KAYAK ROWS L/R
C2. CABLE/ROPE LAT PUSH-DOWNS
4 sets x 10 reps (3010) - rest 60s
(3s lower - 0 - 1s lift - 0)
Rest after C2.

D. CABLE/ROPE 3-WAY FACE PULLS
4 sets x 10, 10, 10 reps (2010) - rest 60s
(2s lower - 0 - 1s pull - 0)
10 reps each to eyes, to neck, to chest; rest.

E. CABLE/HANDLE TRANSVERSE ROWS (L/R)
10, 10, 10, 6, 6, 6 reps - rest 45s

BACK ATTACK

★ ★ ★ ★ ★

A: BARBELL PENDLAY ROWS

1. With the barbell on the floor, grip the bar with your hands
   a bit wider than shoulder-width apart.
2. Keep your back parallel to the floor, and pull with your arms.
3. Lower the barbell back to the floor to a dead stop.
4. Repeat.

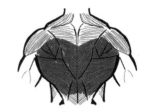

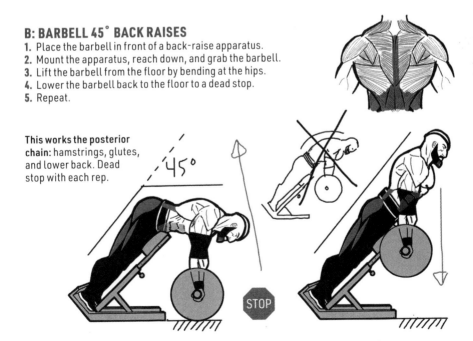

DEAD STOP WITH EACH REP

B: BARBELL 45° BACK RAISES

1. Place the barbell in front of a back-raise apparatus.
2. Mount the apparatus, reach down, and grab the barbell.
3. Lift the barbell from the floor by bending at the hips.
4. Lower the barbell back to the floor to a dead stop.
5. Repeat.

This works the posterior chain: hamstrings, glutes, and lower back. Dead stop with each rep.

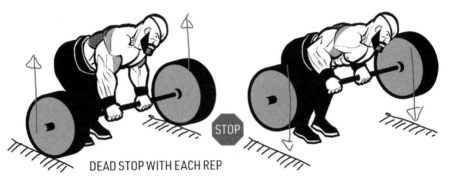

BACK ATTACK

★ ★ ★ ★ ★

C1: CABLE/ROPE KAYAK ROWS (L/R)

1. Attach the rope to a cable machine set at eye level.
2. Grab the rope with a staggered grip, one hand higher than the other.
3. Pull down the rope, keeping your arms extended in a rowing motion, only hinging at the shoulders.
4. Bring the lower hand down to your thighs.
5. Lower the weight.
6. Repeat.
7. Switch sides.

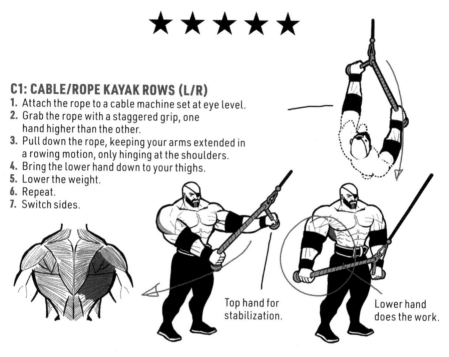

Top hand for stabilization.

Lower hand does the work.

C2: CABLE/ROPE LAT PUSH-DOWNS

1. Attach the rope to a cable machine set at eye level.
2. Grab the rope with your hands and walk back, keeping the cable taut.
3. Drop your hips with your arms extended.
4. Pull down the rope by bending at the hips and pull the rope toward your thighs.
5. Lower the weight by bending at the hips.
6. Repeat.

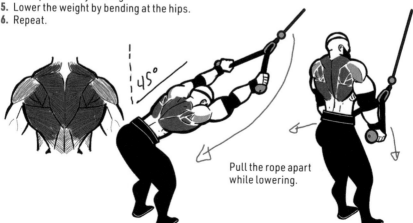

45°

Pull the rope apart while lowering.

BACK ATTACK

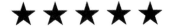

D: CABLE/ROPE 3-WAY FACE PULLS

1. Attach the rope to the cable machine and set it at eye level.
2. Grab the rope with your hands and walk it back, keeping the cable taut.
3. Pull the rope toward your eyes while pulling the rope apart by bending at the elbows.
4. Lower the weight by relaxing your arms.
5. Repeat for 10 reps.
6. Perform a face-pull to your neck for 10 reps.
7. Perform a face-pull to your lower chest for 10 reps.
8. Rest.

TIP: Pull towards the muscle you want to target.

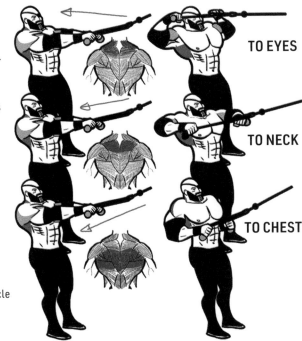

TO EYES

TO NECK

TO CHEST

E: CABLE/HANDLE TRANSVERSE ROWS (L/R)

1. Attach handle to the bottom of the cable machine.
2. Crouch down and place your hand on your thigh for support.
3. Twist your body perpendicular to the cable machine.
4. Grab the handle and pull it across your body.
5. Lower the weight.
6. Repeat.
7. Switch sides.

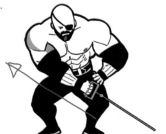

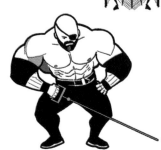

ARM-DAY BLASTER

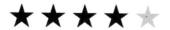

A. BARBELL BICEPS CURLS (STRIP SETS)
4 sets x 8, 8, 8 reps - rest 60s
E.g.: 10 reps x 80 lbs, 60 lbs, 40 lbs

B. TRICEPS DIPS (BODYWEIGHT)
5 sets x 8 reps (5010) - rest 45s
(5s lower - 0 - 1s lift - 0)
Keep your chest upright.

C1. DB LYING BICEPS CURLS
C2. DB OVERHEAD TRICEPS PRESS (SUPERSET)
4 sets x 10 reps (2010) - rest 60s
(2s lower - 0 - 1s curl/lift - 0)
Perform C1 and then C2. Rest. Repeat.

D. BB SKULL CRUSHERS
4 sets x 8 reps - rest 60s
Warm-up sets don't count.

E. DB HAMMER CURLS (RUN RACK UP)
6+ sets x 8–5 reps - rest 30s
Start light and build up. Increase 5 lbs/set.

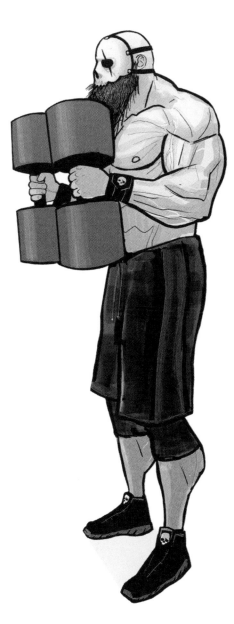

ARM-DAY BLASTER

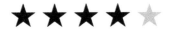

A: BARBELL BICEPS CURLS

1. Grip the barbell with a supine (palm-up) grip about shoulder-width apart.
2. Bend at the elbows to curl the barbell up while keeping your elbows tucked in.
3. Lower the barbell.
4. Repeat.
5. Avoid body English and cheating the weight up.

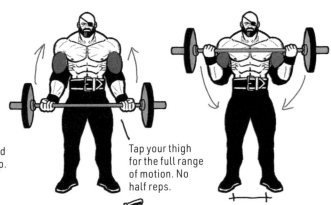

Tap your thigh for the full range of motion. No half reps.

Stand with your feet shoulder-width apart in "strong position." You're not a ballerina.

VARIATION: Mix up biceps curls by using straight and EZ-Curl bars.

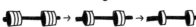

A strip set or drop set is made up of multiple sets of decreasing resistance. Muscle fibers will fatigue, but reducing the resistance enables more work. Strip sets can be performed by taking off single plates or percentage drops.

B: TRICEPS DIPS

1. Step up to or position yourself on a dip apparatus.
2. Start with extended arms and supporting your bodyweight.
3. Lower yourself by bending at your elbows.
4. Keep your chest up and your feet back.
5. Lift yourself by extending your arms.
6. Repeat.

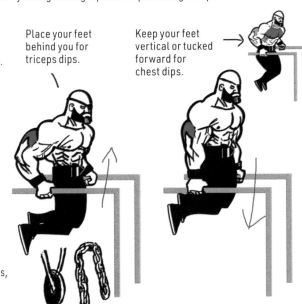

Place your feet behind you for triceps dips.

Keep your feet vertical or tucked forward for chest dips.

VARIATION: Too easy? Add a weight belt or chains, or use a slower tempo.

ARM-DAY BLASTER

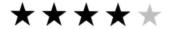

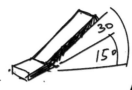

C1: DB LYING BICEPS CURLS

1. Adjust an incline bench to an angle of 15–30°.
2. Grab the dumbbells and lie back on the bench.
3. Let your arms hang off the bench.
4. With a supine (palm-up) grip, bend at the elbows to curl the dumbbells up.
5. Squeeze at the top.
6. Lower the dumbbells.
7. Repeat for reps.

Your prone positioning on the bench eliminates any cheating or momentum through the hips.

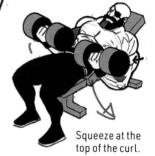

Avoid using your shoulders to lift by keeping your shoulders back.

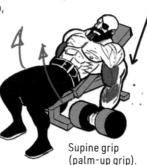

Supine grip (palm-up grip).

Squeeze at the top of the curl.

C2: DB OVERHEAD TRICEPS PRESS

1. Grab one dumbbell and lift it overhead.
2. Position the dumbbell behind your head with bent elbows.
3. Extend your arms and lift the dumbbell up.
4. Lower in a controlled manner by bending your elbows.
5. Repeat for reps.

TIP: Standing will engage more of your core than when you are seated.

This press allows for your elbows to flare out, whereas with extensions, the elbows point forward.

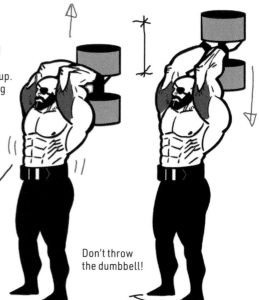

Don't throw the dumbbell!

Keep your feet shoulder-width apart.

ARM-DAY BLASTER

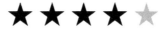

D: BB SKULL CRUSHERS

1. Start seated, with the barbell on your lap.
2. Lie back and press the bar upward, with your arms extended.
3. Lower the bar toward your forehead by bending at the elbows.
4. Repeat.
5. When finished, lower the barbell to your chest and sit up.

VARIATIONS: Use EZ-Curl or hammer-curl bars, which are easier on your wrists.

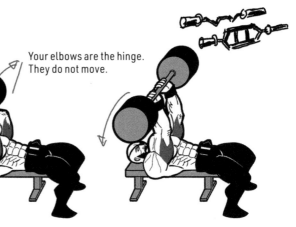

Your elbows are the hinge. They do not move.

E: DB HAMMER CURLS

1. Start with the dumbbells to your side with a hammer (or neutral) grip.
2. Bend at the elbows to curl the dumbbells up while keeping the elbows tucked in.
3. Lower the weight.
4. Repeat.
5. Avoid swinging and using momentum.

"Run rack up" refers to the set method of increasing the dumbbell weight by 5–10 lbs per set.

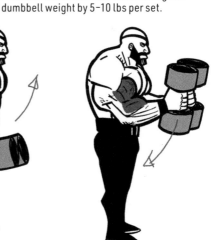

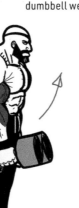

In a neutral grip (hammer grip), the palms face each other.

NINE STAGES OF HELL: PLATES

Complete the 9 exercises as a big circuit.

15s rest between exercises. Rest 60s after A9.

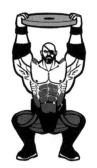 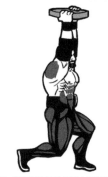 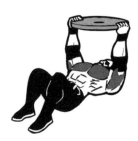

| A1. OVERHEAD SQUAT | A2. OVERHEAD LUNGE | A3. FLOOR CHEST PRESS |

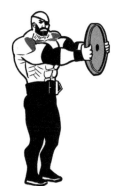 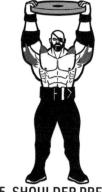 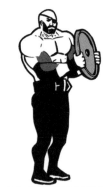

| A4. FRONT RAISE | A5. SHOULDER PRESS | A6. BICEPS CURL |

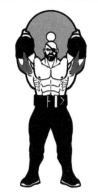 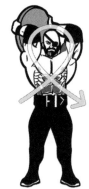 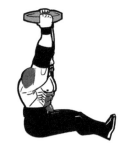

| A7. TRICEPS EXTENSION | A8. RIBBON | A9. COFFIN SIT-UP |

VARIATIONS: Replace with dumbbells or kettlebells, change work time to 15–20 reps, or mix up the exercise order.

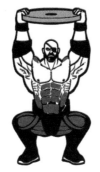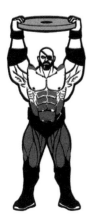

A1: OVERHEAD SQUAT

1. Raise the weight above your head.
2. Stand with your legs wider than shoulder-width apart.
3. Keep your torso upright, and squat down while the weight stays above your head.
4. Squat up and repeat.

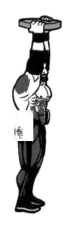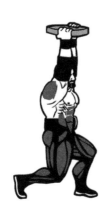

A2: OVERHEAD LUNGE

1. Raise the weight above your head.
2. Stand with your feet together.
3. Keep your torso upright, and step forward into a lunge.
4. Perform as walking lunges or standing alternating lunges.

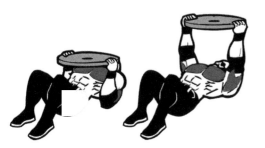

A3: FLOOR CHEST PRESS

1. Lie on the floor with the weight on your chest and your elbows by your side.
2. Extend your arms upward and raise the weight above your chest.
3. Lower back to the starting position and repeat.

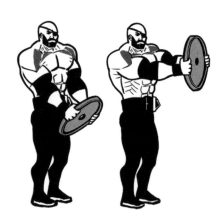

A4: FRONT RAISE

1. Start by holding the weight at your thighs.
2. Keep your arms extended, and raise the weight to shoulder height.
3. Lower your weight back to the starting position and repeat.

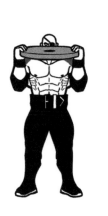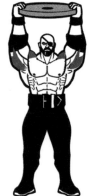

A5: SHOULDER PRESS

1. Start with the weight at shoulder height.
2. Extend your arms up over your head.
3. Lower your arms back to the starting position and repeat.

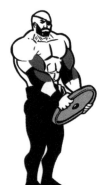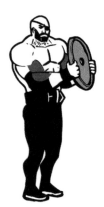

A6: BICEPS CURL

1. Start by holding the weight at your thighs.
2. Bend only at the elbows, and raise the weight.
3. Lower the weight back to the starting position and repeat.

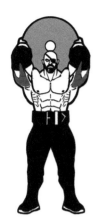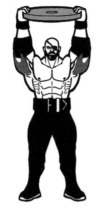

A7: TRICEPS EXTENSION
1. Raise the weight above your head with your arms extended.
2. Bend at the elbows, and lower the weight behind your head.
3. Raise the weight to the starting position and repeat.

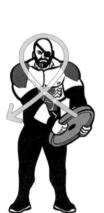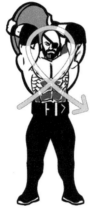

A8: RIBBON
1. Start by holding the weight with extended arms by your thigh.
2. Raise the weight over and around the opposite shoulder.
3. Move the weight behind your head to the other shoulder, lower to the opposite thigh, and repeat.

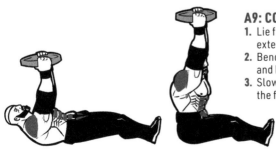

A9: COFFIN SIT-UP
1. Lie flat on the floor with your arms extended, holding the weight.
2. Bend at the hips to raise your torso and keep your arms extended above.
3. Slowly lower your back to the floor and repeat.

GLUTE HAM SAMMICH

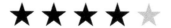

A. LAYING LEG CURLS (WARM UP)
5 sets x 20 reps - rest 30s
(30% 1RM)

B. BARBELL 45°
BACK RAISES
10, 10, 5, 5, 3, 3, 3 reps - rest 60s
Reset/pause at bottom.

C. BARBELL SQUATS
3 sets x 3 reps - rest 120s
Build up to 3 reps max.

D. BB ROMANIAN DEADLIFTS
4 sets x 8 reps (4010) - rest 60s
(4s lower - 0 - 1s lift - 0)
Lower bar to mid shin.

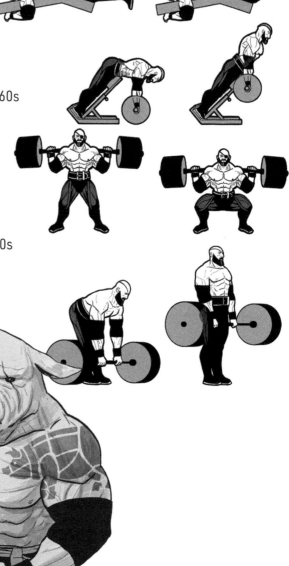

GLUTE HAM SAMMICH

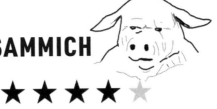

★★★★☆

A. LAYING LEG CURLS (WARM-UP)
Warm up the hamstrings
before your big lifts.
· 100 total reps of light weight.

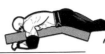

Keep the
muscle in
stretch at
bottom of rep.

Full range
of motion.

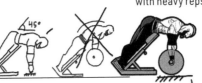

Warm-up sets of 5 sets x 20 reps
or 4 sets x 25 reps.

B. BARBELL 45° BACK RAISES
Work your posterior chain:
glutes, hamstrings, low back.
· Increase your deadlift.

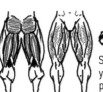

Warm up with your
bodyweight tapping
the ground.

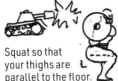

Rest the bar on the floor
with heavy reps.

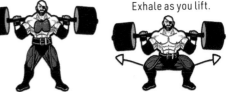

Don't round
your back.

C. BARBELL SQUATS
Warm-up sets will prepare your
body for heavier loads.
· Always leave 1 rep in the tank.

Take a deep breath
at the top of the
lift for bracing.

Exhale as you lift.

Squat so that
your thighs are
parallel to the floor.

Drive the knees out.

D. BB ROMANIAN DEADLIFTS
Keep narrow foot stance.
· Open up the feet a bit for
  more glute activation.
· Start from the floor.
· Don't waste energy by
  unracking the weight off a
  rack and then walking out.

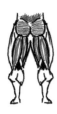

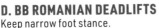

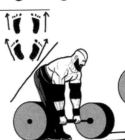

Stop 2 inches
from the floor.

No pause at the top,
to keep tension on
the glutes (optional).

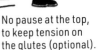

DREAD THE SLED

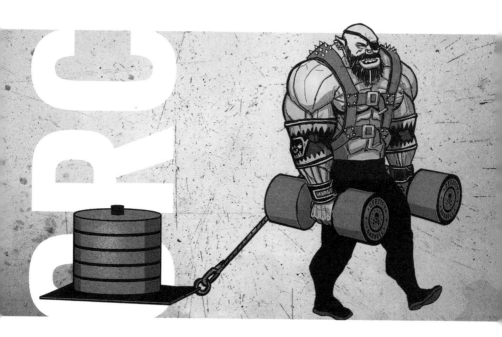

A1. SLED HARNESS PULL—FORWARD
A2. SLED HARNESS PULL—BACKWARD
3 sets x 50 ft, 50 ft - rest 60s
50 ft forward, 50 ft backward

B. SLED HARNESS PULL WITH DB CARRY
3 sets x 100 ft - rest 60s
Pull bodyweight + 80 lbs (2 x 40-lb DB)

C. SLED ONE ARM ROWS (L/R)
3 sets x 10 reps - rest 60s

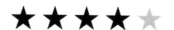

DREAD THE SLED

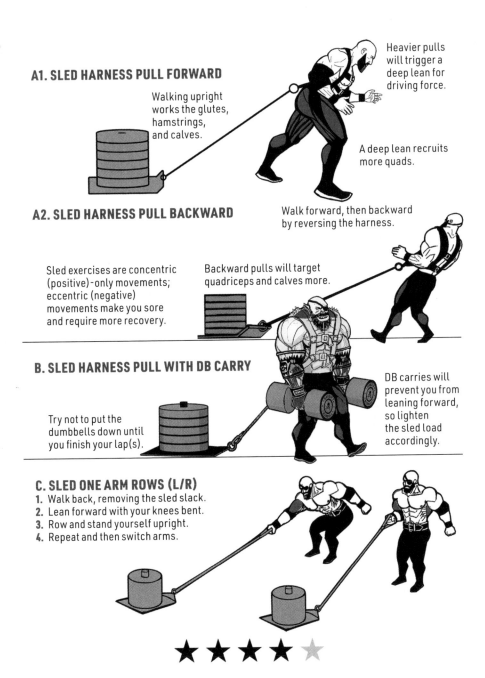

A1. SLED HARNESS PULL FORWARD

Heavier pulls will trigger a deep lean for driving force.

Walking upright works the glutes, hamstrings, and calves.

A deep lean recruits more quads.

A2. SLED HARNESS PULL BACKWARD

Walk forward, then backward by reversing the harness.

Sled exercises are concentric (positive)-only movements; eccentric (negative) movements make you sore and require more recovery.

Backward pulls will target quadriceps and calves more.

B. SLED HARNESS PULL WITH DB CARRY

DB carries will prevent you from leaning forward, so lighten the sled load accordingly.

Try not to put the dumbbells down until you finish your lap(s).

C. SLED ONE ARM ROWS (L/R)
1. Walk back, removing the sled slack.
2. Lean forward with your knees bent.
3. Row and stand yourself upright.
4. Repeat and then switch arms.

★ ★ ★ ★ ☆

BACK-BEEF BASICS

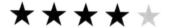

A. BARBELL DEADLIFTS (SUMO)
3 sets x 2 reps - rest 120s
Sumo or conventional.

B. BB PENDLAY ROWS
3 sets x 5 reps - rest 60s
Tap the ground with each rep.

C. CHEST-SUPPORTED BB ROWS
4 sets x 20 reps - rest 45s
Pull into the bench.

D. PULL-UPS/CHIN-UPS
100 total reps
Mix up your grip.

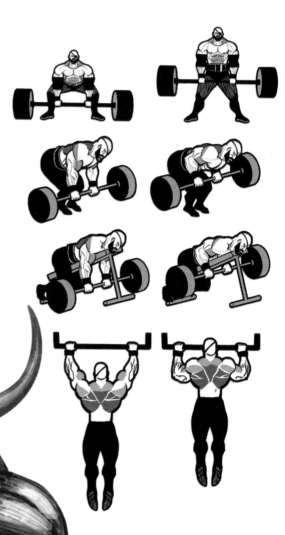

LEG KILLER

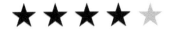

A. BARBELL BOX SQUATS
4 sets x 5 reps (3111) - rest 60s
· (3s lower - 1s pause on box - 1s lift - 1s pause at top)

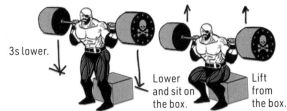

3s lower.

Lower and sit on the box.

Lift from the box.

B. MACHINE LEG PRESS SINGLE LEG (L/R)
4 sets x 10 reps - rest 60s

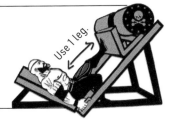
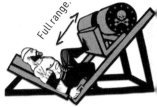

Use 1 leg.

Full range.

C1. MACHINE LEG CURLS
C2. MACHINE LEG EXTENSIONS
4 sets x 10 reps (2010) - rest 60s
· (2s lower - 0 - 1s lift - 0)
· No rest between C1 and C2.

The slower negative makes lowering reps more difficult. More work = more growth.

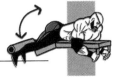
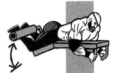

2s lower.

D. SLED PULLS–WALKING PACE (OR PROWLER PUSH)
1 set x 20 laps
· (60% bodyweight)
· 1 lap = 50 ft

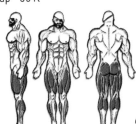

20-lap walk. Continuous laps. No breaks.

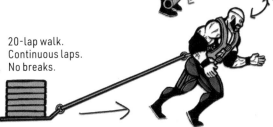

CRAZY EIGHTS

★ ★ ★ ★ ☆

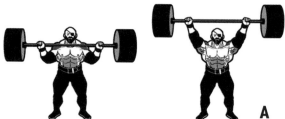

A. BB SHOULDER PRESS
4 sets x 8 reps - rest 60s

A

B. DB SHOULDER PRESS
4 sets x 8 reps - rest 60s

C. DB GIANT SHOULDER SET
4 sets x 8 reps - rest 60s

C1. DB Y-PRESS
C2. DB SIDE LATERAL RAISES
C3. DB BENT-OVER REVERSE FLYES
C4. DB HERCULES PUNCH
Perform C1, C2, C3, C4 - rest 60s
Use lighter weight.

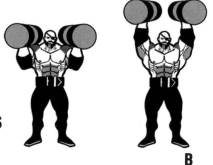

B

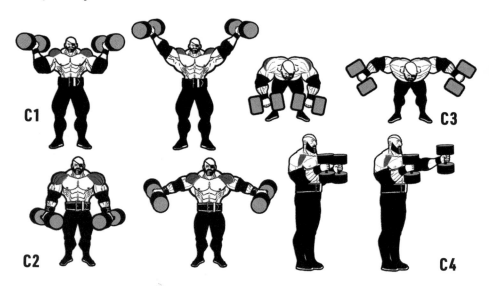

C1

C2

C3

C4

LANDMINE SUPERSET

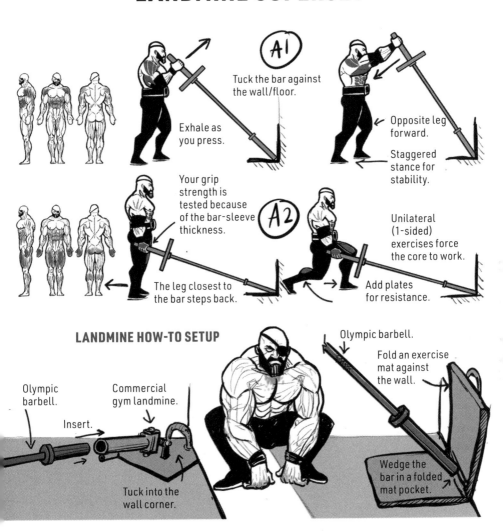

A1

Tuck the bar against the wall/floor.

Exhale as you press.

Opposite leg forward.

Staggered stance for stability.

Your grip strength is tested because of the bar-sleeve thickness.

A2

Unilateral (1-sided) exercises force the core to work.

The leg closest to the bar steps back.

Add plates for resistance.

LANDMINE HOW-TO SETUP

Olympic barbell.

Insert.

Commercial gym landmine.

Tuck into the wall corner.

Olympic barbell.

Fold an exercise mat against the wall.

Wedge the bar in a folded mat pocket.

A1. LANDMINE SHOULDER PRESS (L/R)
A2. LANDMINE REVERSE LUNGE (L/R)
4 sets x 8 reps (2010) - rest 60s
(2s lower - 0 - 1s lift - 0)

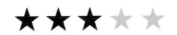

★ ★ ★ ☆ ☆

BEYOND DELTS

★ ★ ★ ☆ ☆

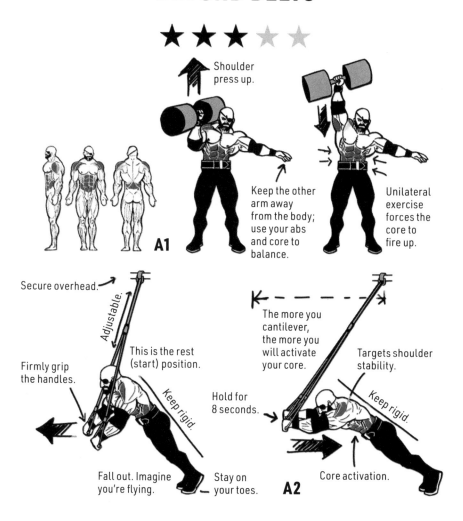

Shoulder press up.

Keep the other arm away from the body; use your abs and core to balance.

A1

Unilateral exercise forces the core to fire up.

Secure overhead.

Adjustable.

Firmly grip the handles.

This is the rest (start) position.

Keep rigid.

Fall out. Imagine you're flying.

Stay on your toes.

The more you cantilever, the more you will activate your core.

Targets shoulder stability.

Hold for 8 seconds.

Keep rigid.

Core activation.

A2

A1. DUMBBELL SHOULDER PRESS (L/R)
5 sets x 6 reps

A2. SUSPENSION TRAINER FALL OUTS
5 sets x 4 reps (1810) - rest 45s
(1s lower - 8s bottom hold - 1s lift - 0)

PLANKS PIZZA SLICES (L/R)

4 sets x 10 reps or 30s
Use 10-lb or 25-lb plate.

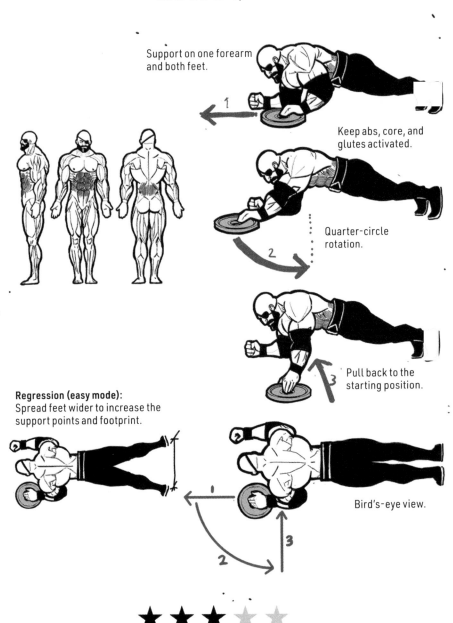

Support on one forearm and both feet.

Keep abs, core, and glutes activated.

Quarter-circle rotation.

Pull back to the starting position.

Regression (easy mode):
Spread feet wider to increase the support points and footprint.

Bird's-eye view.

★ ★ ★ ☆ ☆

VALHALLA CIRCUIT

★ ★ ★ ★ ★

4-Round Circuit
45s work/15s rest per exercise

A1. KETTLEBELL (KB) SQUATS
A2. PUSH-UPS
A3. KB ALTERNATING ROWS
A4. KB RUSSIAN TWISTS
A1, A2, A3, A4, rest 60s
Can substitute work time with 20 reps.

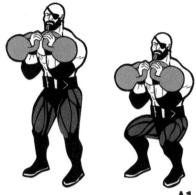

A1

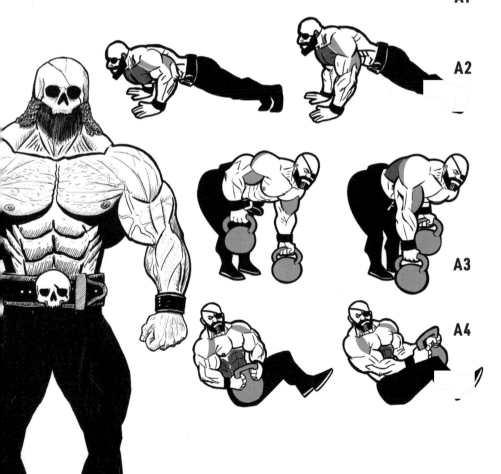

A2

A3

A4

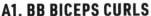

A1. BB BICEPS CURLS

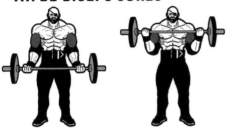

A2. BB BENT-OVER TRICEPS KICKBACKS

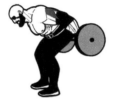

A3. DB BICEPS CURLS

A4. DB OVERHEAD TRICEPS EXTENSIONS

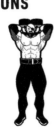

BIG PIPES

4-Round Circuit
45s work/15s rest per exercise
A1, A2, A3, A4, rest 60s
Use same BB weight: A1 and A2.
Use same DB weight: A3 and A4.

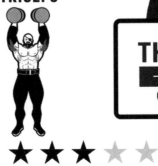

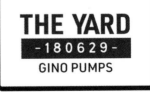

THE YARD
-180629-
GINO PUMPS

★ ★ ★ ★ ★

A1. BB CLEAN AND PRESS

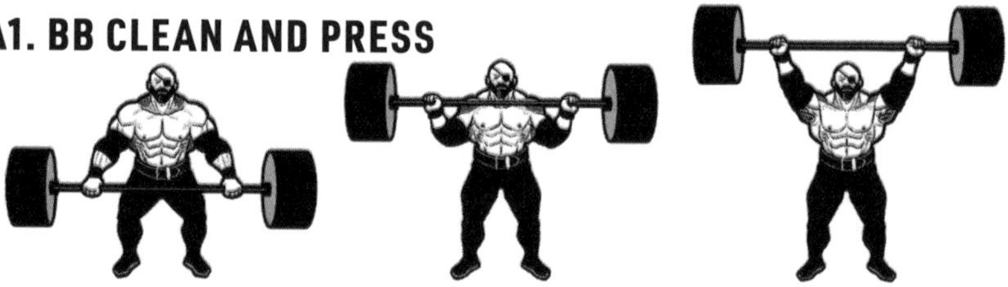

A2. BB PENDLAY ROWS

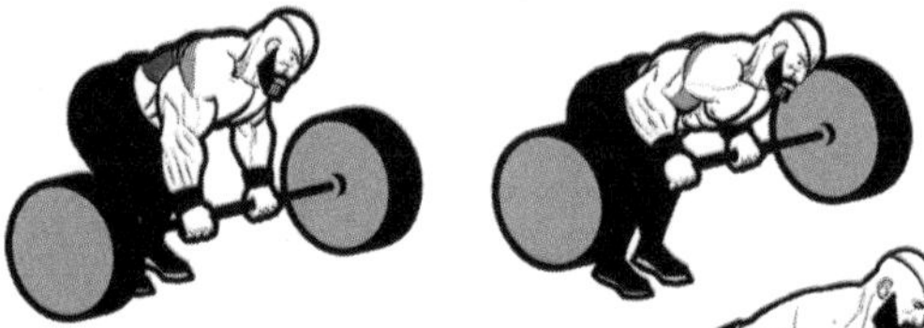

A3. STIFF-LEG DEADLIFTS

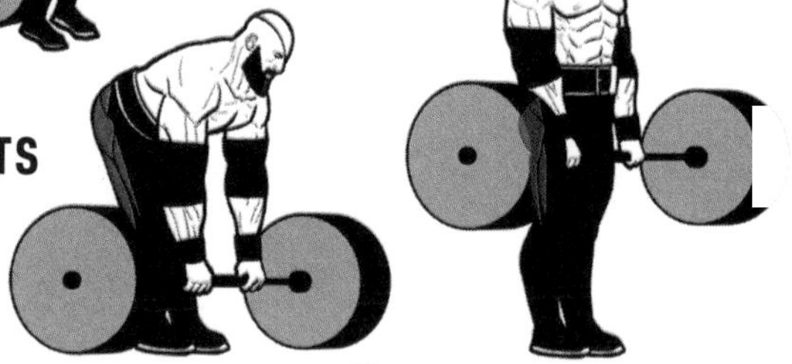

A4. PUSH-UPS

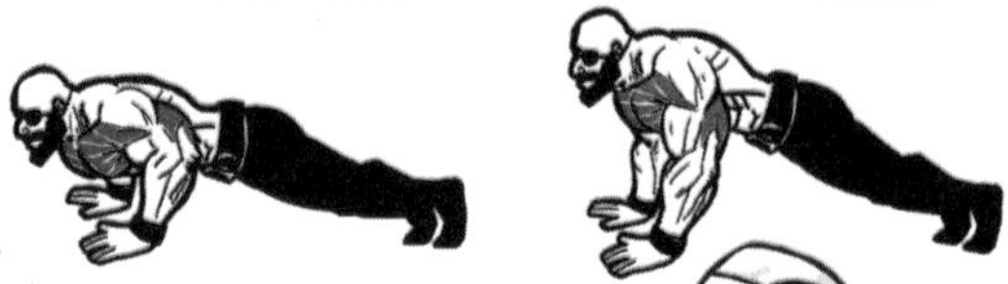

YARD WORK

4-Round Circuit
45s work/15s rest per exercise
A1, A2, A3, A4, rest 60s
Use the same weight throughout.

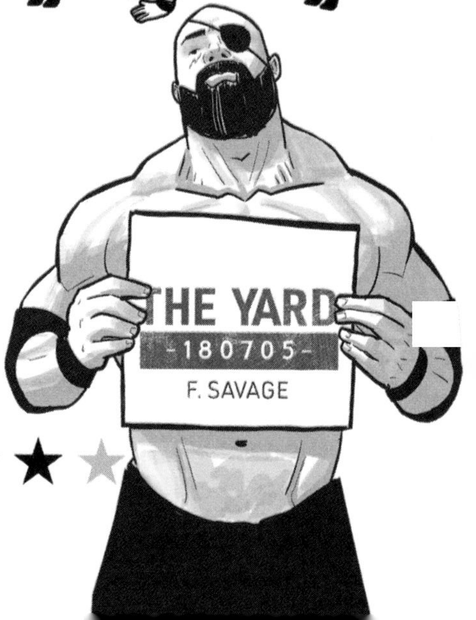

THE YARD
-180705-
F. SAVAGE

★★★★☆

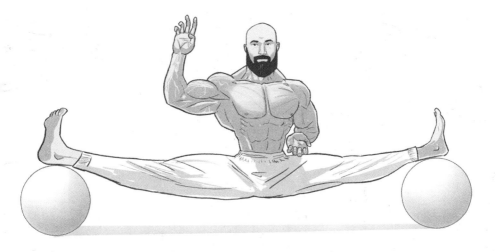

STRETCHES

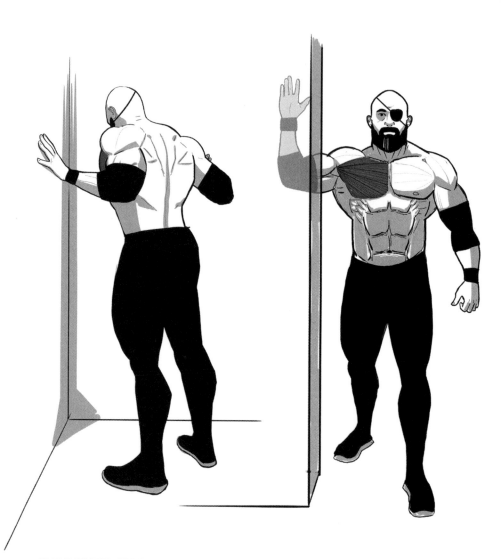

CORNER WALL STRETCH

1. Stand near a wall corner.
2. Place your hands against the walls, with your elbows bent in push-up position.
3. Lean forward gently.
4. Hold for 10 to 30 seconds.

WALL CHEST STRETCH

1. Raise your arm to shoulder height against a wall.
2. Bend your elbow and point your hand to the ceiling.
3. Rotate your torso slowly away from your hand.
4. Hold for 10 to 30 seconds.
5. Repeat for the other side.

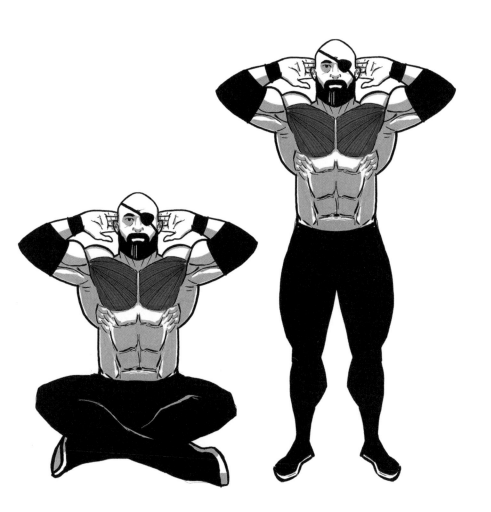

CHEST EXPANSION

1. Raise your elbows to shoulder height, with your fingers near your ears.
2. Pull your elbows back and squeeze your shoulder blades.
3. Hold for 10 to 30 seconds.

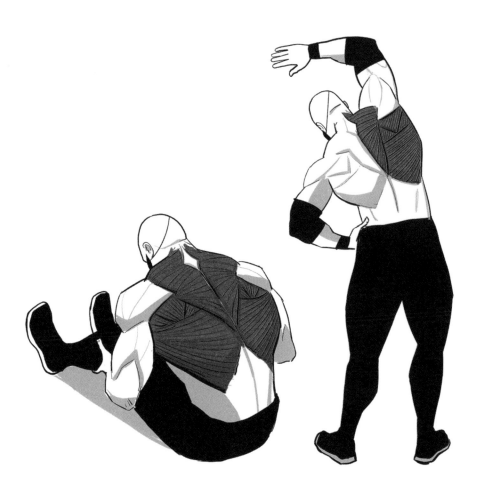

UPPER BACK SCOOP

1. While seated, bend your knees and reach for your thighs.
2. Grasp your thighs and round your upper back.
3. Hold for 10 to 30 seconds.

BACK SIDE REACH

1. Stand with your feet shoulder-width apart.
2. Place one hand on your hip, and raise one hand above your head. Lean to the opposite side.
3. Hold for 10 to 30 seconds.
4. Repeat for the other side.

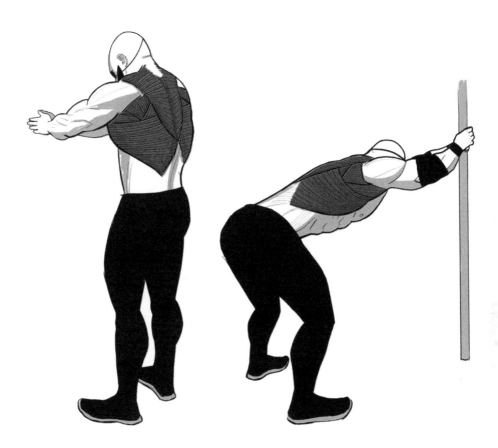

BACK FRONT REACH

1. Raise your hands to chest height in front of your body.
2. Place your hands together.
3. Reach forward with your hands.
4. Hold for 10 to 30 seconds.

POLE STRETCH

1. Stand with your feet shoulder-width apart.
2. Grab a pole or support with both hands.
3. Lean your body to one side.
4. Hold for 10 to 30 seconds.
5. Repeat for the other side.

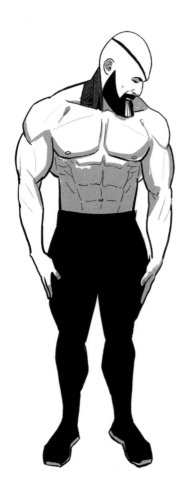

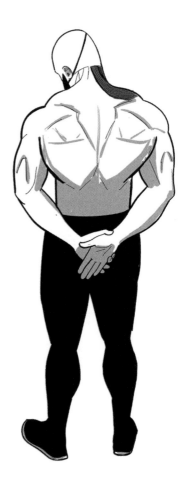

CHIN DROP

1. Keep your arms at your sides.
2. Drop your chin diagonally toward your upper chest.
3. Hold for 10 to 30 seconds.
4. Repeat for the other side.

HEAD TILT

1. Clasp your hands behind your body.
2. Tilt your head to one side.
3. Hold for 10 to 30 seconds.
4. Repeat for the other side.

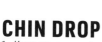

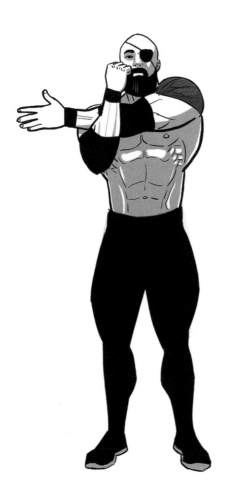

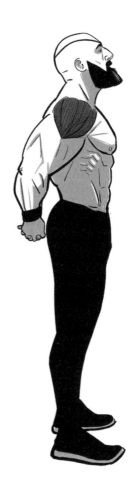

ARM CROSS

1. Raise your arm to shoulder height and across your torso.
2. Use your other hand to pull your arm close to your torso.
3. Hold for 10 to 30 seconds.
4. Repeat for the other side.

ARMS BEHIND

1. Stand with your feet shoulder-width apart.
2. Clasp your hands together behind your back.
3. Lift your hands upward.
4. Hold for 10 to 30 seconds.

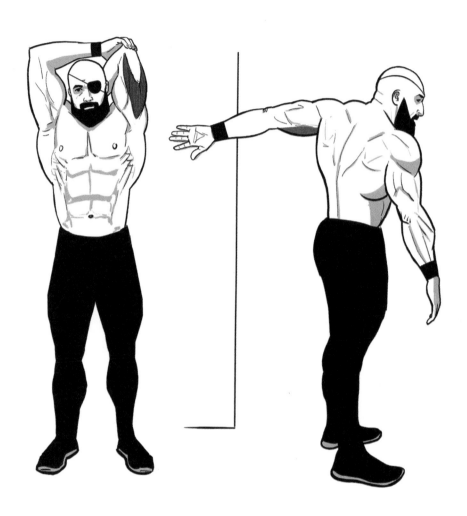

TRICEPS STRETCH

1. Raise one arm above your head.
2. Bend your forearm and reach toward your shoulder blades.
3. Use your other hand to gently push your elbow.
4. Hold for 10 to 30 seconds.
5. Repeat for the other side.

BICEPS STRETCH

1. Raise your arm to shoulder height against the wall.
2. Position the back of your hand with the thumb down.
3. Slowly rotate your torso away from the hand.
4. Hold for 10 to 30 seconds.
5. Repeat for the other side.

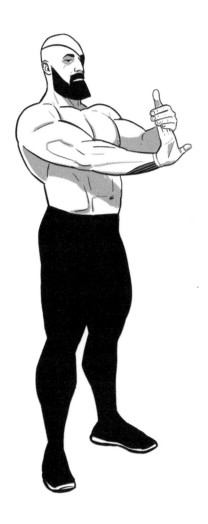
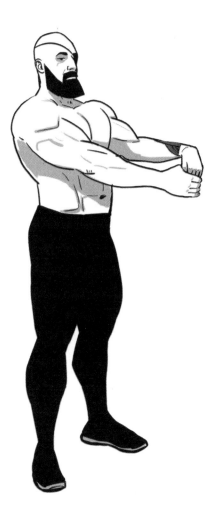

WRIST EXTEND

1. Extend one arm forward with the palm facing forward.
2. Use the other hand to gently pull back, extending the wrist.
3. Hold for 10 to 30 seconds.
4. Repeat for the other side.

WRIST FLEX

1. Extend one arm forward with the palm facing down.
2. Use the other hand to gently pull down, flexing the wrist.
3. Hold for 10 to 30 seconds.
4. Repeat for the other side.

SIDE OBLIQUE STRETCH

1. Stand with your feet shoulder-width apart.
2. Place one hand on your hip, and raise the other hand above your head. Lean to the opposite side.
3. Hold for 10 to 30 seconds.
4. Repeat for the other side.

COBRA STRETCH

1. Lie flat on the floor with your hands by your shoulders.
2. Raise your chest and abs by pushing up from the floor with your hands.
3. Hold for 10 to 30 seconds.

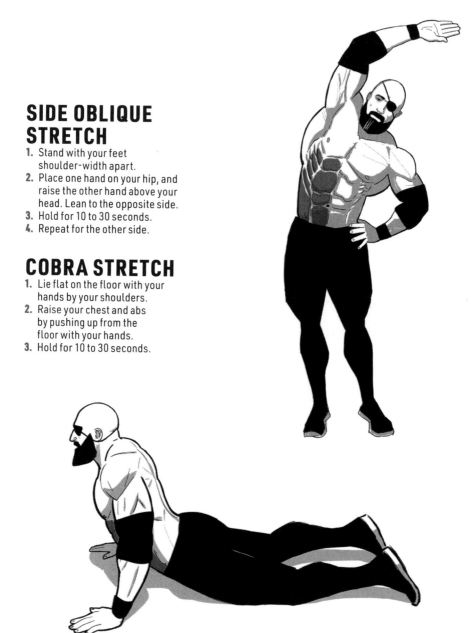

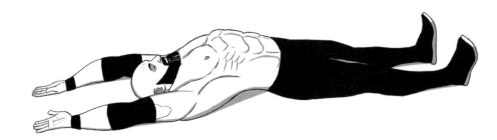

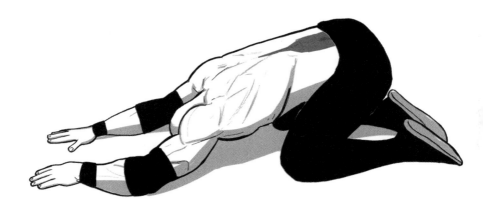

SUPINE ARCH

1. Lie flat on the ground with your hands extended above your head.
2. Reach with your hands away from your body.
3. Gently raise your ribs and lower your back off the ground.
4. Hold for 10 to 30 seconds.

CHILD'S POSE

1. Kneel on the floor on your hands and knees.
2. Sit back and lower your hips onto your heels.
3. Spread your knees out and bring your torso into your thighs.
4. Lay your hands forward, and touch your forehead to the floor.
5. Hold for 10 to 30 seconds.

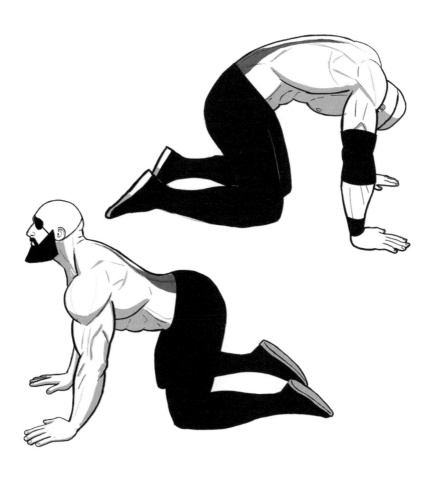

COW STRETCH

1. Start with your hands and knees on the floor.
2. Push your chin up, curl your spine, and push your chest upward.
3. Relax to the starting position.
4. Repeat for 10 repetitions.

CAT STRETCH

1. Start with your hands and knees on the floor.
2. Tuck your chin to your chest, round your spine, and pull your abs inward.
3. Relax to the starting position.
4. Repeat for 10 repetitions.

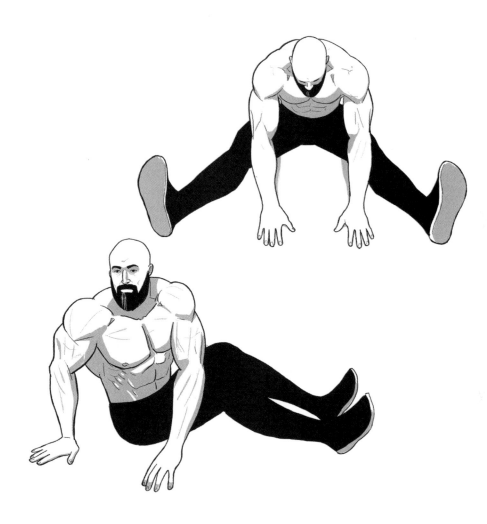

SEATED TWIST

1. Sit on the floor with your knees slightly bent.
2. Twist your torso to one side, and place your hands on the floor.
3. Hold for 10 to 30 seconds.
4. Repeat for the other side.

SEATED REACH

1. Sit on the floor with your legs spread open.
2. Reach forward with your hands on the floor.
3. Hold for 10 to 30 seconds.

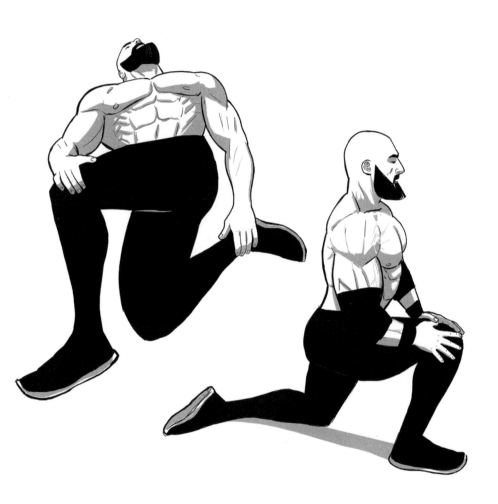

BRETTZEL

1. Lie flat on the ground.
2. Cross one leg over the other thigh.
3. Pull your knee toward your chest with the opposing hand.
4. Grab the other ankle with the other hand.
5. Hold for 10 to 30 seconds.
6. Repeat for the other side.

KNEELING LUNGE

1. Kneel on the ground, keeping the torso upright.
2. Place your hands on one leg and gently lean forward.
3. Hold for 10 to 30 seconds.
4. Repeat for the other side.

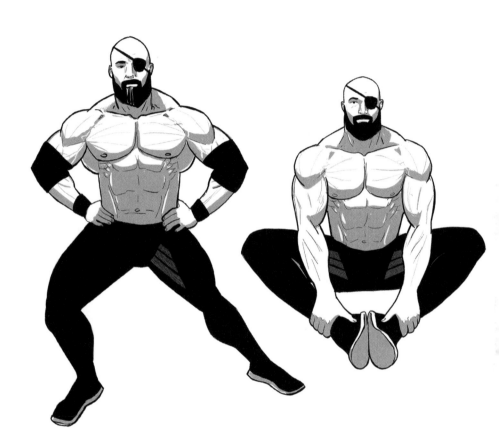

SIDE LUNGE

1. Start in a wide stance with your hands on your hips.
2. Lunge to one side while keeping the other leg straight.
3. Keep your torso upright.
4. Hold for 10 to 30 seconds.
5. Repeat for the other side.

BUTTERFLY STRETCH

1. While seated, bring the soles of your feet together.
2. Use your elbows to gently push your thighs against the floor.
3. Hold for 10 to 30 seconds.

QUAD STRETCH

1. Place one hand on the wall for support.
2. Bend the other leg, and grasp your lower leg.
3. Hold for 10 to 30 seconds.
4. Repeat for the other side.

HURDLER'S STRETCH

1. Lie on your side and support your head with your hand.
2. Keep one leg extended, and bend the other leg.
3. Grab the bent leg near the ankle.
4. Hold for 10 to 30 seconds.
5. Repeat for the other side.

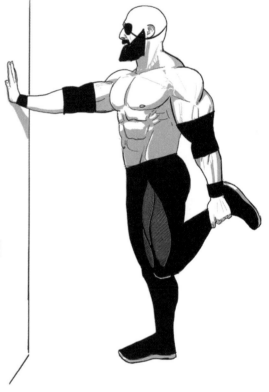

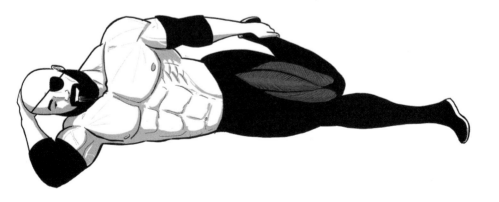

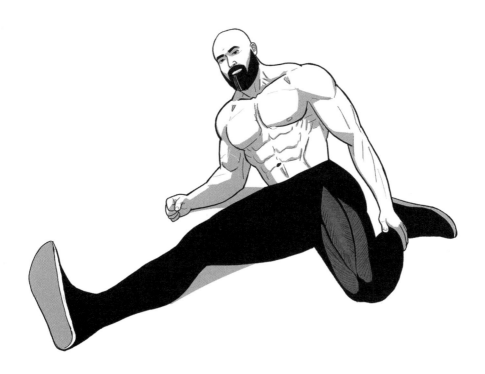

BACK FRONT REACH

1. Sit on the floor, and extend one leg out.
2. Bend the other leg back.
3. Lean to the opposite side.
4. Hold the stretch for 15 to 30 seconds.
5. Repeat for the other side.

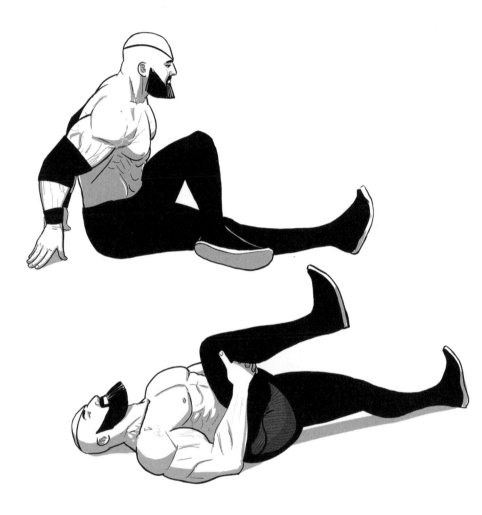

SEATED LEG CROSS

1. Cross one leg over the other leg while seated on the floor.
2. Place your hands behind you, and gently push your torso forward.
3. Hold for 10 to 30 seconds.
4. Repeat for the other side.

LEG HUG

1. Lie flat on the ground with your legs extended.
2. Bend one knee, and grab that leg with your hands.
3. Gently pull toward your chest.
4. Hold for 10 to 30 seconds.
5. Repeat for the other side.

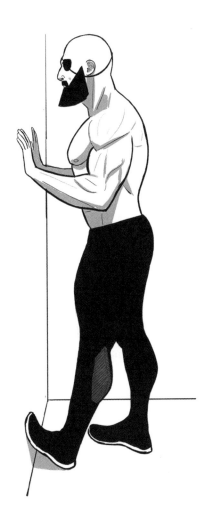

CALF WALL STRETCH

1. Place your hands on the wall for support.
2. Press the toes of one foot against the
   wall, and push your heel into the ground.
3. Hold for 10 to 30 seconds.
4. Repeat for the other side.

EIGHT-WEEK WORKOUT PLAN

For those who are looking for a specific plan or customized regimen to try, what follows is an eight-week workout program. The more work you put into it, the better the results you'll see. What's more, with this plan, you won't be overwhelmed with hundreds of exercises. These are just basics that, if done correctly, are proven to work.

THE INSTRUCTIONS FOR FOLLOWING THIS PLAN ARE SIMPLE, THOUGH NOT EASY:

1. Try to do four workouts in a week. To help you achieve this, I've come up with a flexible weekly two-day system. Perform each workout twice a week. If you'd like to train another day, then mix it up with some other exercises from the book.
2. Trust the plan. Although the week-to-week changes are subtle, they are vital.
3. Get seven or eight hours of sleep every night. Recovery is important.
4. Eat cleaner, and drink plenty of water.
5. You can substitute some of the exercises with variations, except for exercises A and B. Those are foundational, compound-strength exercises and are nonnegotiable. The first two exercises at the beginning of the workout will measure your progress and gains. There is a method to the madness.
6. It will be helpful to document your weight and measurements and to take full front, back, and side photos the day prior to your first workout. At the end of the program (i.e., after eight weeks), document your weight and measurements once again and take new photos. Compare the starting and ending data.
7. Keep a workout journal or have your A and B exercise numbers ready for your workout. A workout journal can be used to track your progress, your strength gains, your mood, your energy, the weights you used, and any other workout notes.
8. Warm-ups are not noted for these workouts, so warm up appropriately and build up to your working sets on exercises A and B (deadlifts, bench press, squats, and shoulder press).
9. Do the work, my friend.

WEEK 1			
WK1-D1			
A	BB Deadlifts	3 sets x 10 reps - rest 60s	(12 rep max)
B	BB Bench Press	3 sets x 10 reps - rest 60s	(12 rep max)
C	BB Pendlay Rows	3 sets x 10 reps - rest 60s	
D	DB Chest Press	3 sets x 10 reps - rest 60s	
E	DB Chest Flyes	3 sets x 10 reps - rest 60s	
F	Pull-Ups	20 total reps	
WK1-D2			
A	BB Shoulder Press	3 sets x 10 reps - rest 60s	(12 rep max)
B	BB Squats	3 sets x 10 reps - rest 60s	(12 rep max)
C	BB Stiff-Leg Deadlifts	3 sets x 10 reps - rest 60s	
D	DB Walking Lunges	3 sets x 20 steps - rest 60s	
E	DB Side Lateral Raises	3 sets x 10 reps - rest 60s	
F	BB Curls	3 sets x 10 reps - rest 60s	
G	Cable/Rope Triceps Push-Downs	3 sets x 10 reps - rest 60s	
WK1- D3	same as WK1-D1	replace Pull-Ups with Chin-Ups	
WK1-D4	same as WK1-D2		

	WEEK 2		
WK2-D1			
A	BB Deadlifts	4 sets x 10 reps - rest 60s	(+10 lbs of WK1-D1 A)
B	BB Bench Press	4 sets x 10 reps - rest 60s	(+10 lbs of WK1-D1 B)
C	Cable/V-Handle Seated Rows	4 sets x 10 reps - rest 60s	(or Machine Rows)
D	Lat Pull-Downs	4 sets x 10 reps - rest 60s	bar, V-handle, or rope
E	DB Incline Chest Press	4 sets x 10 reps - rest 60s	
F	DB Incline Chest Flyes	4 sets x 10 reps - rest 60s	
G	Pull-Ups	25 total reps	
WK2-D2			
A	BB Shoulder Press	4 sets x 10 reps - rest 60s	(+10 lbs of WK1-D2 A)
B	BB Squats	4 sets x 10 reps - rest 60s	(+10 lbs of WK1-D2 B)
C	DB Farmer's Walk	3 sets x 100 ft - rest 90s	(80% bodyweight)
D	Machine Leg Press	3 sets x 10 reps - rest 60s	
E	DB Front Raises	4 sets x 10 reps - rest 60s	
F	DB Curls	4 sets x 10 reps - rest 60s	
G	DB Triceps Overhead Press	4 sets x 10 reps - rest 60s	
WK2-D3	same as WK2-D1	replace Pull-Ups with Chin-Ups	
WK2-D4	same as WK2-D2		

WEEK 3			
WK3-D1			
A	BB Deadlifts	5 sets x 8 reps - rest 60s	(+10 lbs of WK2-D1 A)
B	BB Bench Press	5 sets x 8 reps - rest 60s	(+10 lbs of WK2-D1 B)
C	BB Pendlay Rows	3 sets x 8 reps - rest 60s	
D	DB Chest Press	3 sets x 8 reps - rest 60s	
E	DB Chest Flyes	3 sets x 8 reps - rest 60s	
F	Pull-Ups	30 total reps	
WK3-D2			
A	BB Shoulder Press	5 sets x 8 reps - rest 60	(+10 lbs of WK2-D2 A)
B	BB Squats	5 sets x 8 reps - rest 60s	(+10 lbs of WK2-D2 B)
C	BB Stiff-Leg Deadlifts	3 sets x 10 reps - rest 60s	
D	DB Walking Lunges—Long Stride	3 sets x 20 steps - rest 60s	Long stride for glutes
E	DB Side Lateral Raises	3 sets x 8 reps - rest 60s	
F	BB Curls	3 sets x 8 reps - rest 60s	
G	Cable/Rope Triceps Push-Downs	3 sets x 8 reps - rest 60s	
WK3-D3	same as WK3-D1	replace Pull-Ups with Chin-Ups	
WK3-D4	same as WK3-D2	replace Lunges with short stride	

WEEK 4			
WK4-D1			
A	BB Deadlifts	3 sets x 6 reps - rest 60s	(+20 lbs of WK3-D1 A)
B	BB Bench Press	3 sets x 6 reps - rest 60s	(+20 lbs of WK3-D1 B)
C	Cable/V-Handle Seated Rows	3 sets x 10 reps - rest 60s	
D	Machine Chest Press	3 sets x 10 reps - rest 60s	Flat or incline
E	Cable/Handle Chest Flyes	3 sets x 10 reps - rest 60s	
F	Pull-Ups	20 total reps	
WK4-D2			
A	BB Shoulder Press	3 sets x 6 reps - rest 60s	(+20 lbs of WK3-D2 A)
B	BB Squats	3 sets x 6 reps - rest 60s	(+20 lbs of WK3-D2 B)
C	DB Farmer's Walk	4 sets x 100 ft - rest 90s	(80% bodyweight)
D	Machine Leg Press	3 sets x 10 reps - rest 60s	
E	DB Standing Shoulder Press	4 sets x 10 reps - rest 60s	
F	DB Curls	3 sets x 10 reps - rest 60s	
G	DB Triceps Overhead Press	3 sets x 10 reps - rest 60s	
WK4-D3	same as WK4-D1	replace Pull-Ups with Chin-Ups	
WK4-D4	same as WK4-D2		

WEEK 5			
WK5-D1			
A	BB Deadlifts	3 sets x 10 reps - rest 60s	(12 rep max)
B	BB Bench Press	3 sets x 10 reps - rest 60s	(12 rep max)
C	BB Pendlay Rows	3 sets x 8 reps - rest 60s	
D1	DB Chest Flyes	3 sets x 10, 10 reps - rest 60s	perform D1 & D2 as set
D2	DB Chest Press		
E	Pull-Ups	30 total reps	
WK5-D2			
A	BB Shoulder Press	3 sets x 10 reps - rest 60s	(12 rep max)
B	BB Squats	3 sets x 10 reps - rest 60s	(12 rep max)
C	45° Back Raises	3 sets x 12 reps - rest 45s	
D	BB Single-Leg Deadlifts (L/R)	3 sets x 10 reps - rest 60s	
E	Cable Side Lateral Raises	3 sets x 10 reps - rest 60s	
F1	Cable/Rope Hammer Curls	3 sets x 10, 10 reps - rest 60s	perform F1 & F2 as set
F2	Cable/Rope Tri Push-Downs		
WK5-D3	same as WK5-D1	replace Pull-Ups with Chin-Ups	
WK5-D4	same as WK5-D2		

WEEK 6

WK6-D1

A	BB Deadlifts	4 sets x 10 reps - rest 60s	(+10 lbs of WK5-D1 A)
B	BB Bench Press	4 sets x 10 reps - rest 60s	(+10 lbs of WK5-D1 B)
C	Lat Pull-Downs—Wide Grip	3 sets x 10 reps - rest 60s	
D	Cable/Rope Lat Push-Downs	3 sets x 10 reps - rest 60s	
E1	DB Incline Chest Flyes	3 sets x 10, 10 reps - rest 60s	perform E1 & E2 as set
E2	DB Incline Chest Press		
F	Pull-Ups	40 total reps	

WK6-D2

A	BB Shoulder Press	4 sets x 10 reps - rest 60s	(+10 lbs of WK5-D2 A)
B	BB Squats	4 sets x 10 reps - rest 60s	(+10 lbs of WK5-D2 B)
C	DB Farmer's Walk	3 sets x 100 ft - rest 90s	(80% bodyweight)
D	Machine Leg Press	3 sets x 10 reps - rest 60s	
E	Cable Front Raises	4 sets x 10 reps (2011) - rest 60s	
F	Cable/Handles Double Biceps Curls	4 sets x 10 reps - rest 60s	
G	BB Skull Crushers	4 sets x 10 reps (2010) - rest 60s	
WK6-D3	same as WK6-D1	replace Pull-Ups with Chin-Ups	
WK6-D4	same as WK6-D2		

WEEK 7			
WK7-D1			
A	BB Deadlifts	5 sets x 8 reps - rest 60s	(+10 lbs of WK6-D1 A)
B	BB Bench Press	5 sets x 8 reps - rest 60s	(+10 lbs of WK6-D1 B)
C	DB Bent-Over Rows (L/R)	3 sets x 10 reps - rest 60s	
D1	DB Chest Flyes	4 sets x 8, 8 reps - rest 60s	perform D1 & D2 as set
D2	DB Chest Press		
E	Pull-Ups	50 total reps	
WK7-D2			
A	BB Shoulder Press	5 sets x 8 reps - rest 60s	(+10 lbs of WK6-D2 A)
B	BB Squats	5 sets x 8 reps - rest 60s	(+10 lbs of WK6-D2 B)
C	45° Back Raises	3 sets x 12 reps - rest 45s	
D	DB Walking Lunges	3 sets x 20 steps - rest 60s	long stride for glutes
E	DB Side Lateral Raises	3 sets x 10 reps - rest 60s	
F	DB Preacher Curls (L/R)	3 sets x 10 reps - rest 60s	
G	Triceps Dips	3 sets x 10 reps - rest 60s	
WK7-D3	same as WK7-D1	replace Pull-Ups with Chin-Ups	
WK7-D4	same as WK7-D2	replace Lunges with short stride	

WEEK 8			
WK8-D1			
A	BB Deadlifts	3 sets x 6 reps - rest 60s	(+20 lbs of WK7-D1 A)
B	BB Bench Press	3 sets x 6 reps - rest 60s	(+20 lbs of WK7-D1 B)
C	Cable/Rope Face Pulls to Neck	4 sets x 10 reps (3010) - rest 60s	
D	Lat Pull-Downs	4 sets x 10 reps (3010) - rest 60s	bar, V-handle, or rope
E	Machine Chest Press	3 sets x 10 reps (3010) - rest 45s	flat or incline
F	Cable/Handle Chest Flyes	3 sets x 10 reps (3010) - rest 45s	any angle
G	Pull-Ups	60 total reps	
WK8-D2			
A	BB Shoulder Press	3 sets x 6 reps - rest 60s	(+20 lbs of WK7-D2 A)
B	BB Squats	3 sets x 6 reps - rest 60s	(+20 lbs of WK7-D2 B)
C	DB Farmer's Walk	4 sets x 100 ft - rest 90s	(80% bodyweight)
D	Machine Leg Press	5 sets x 20 reps - rest 60s	
E	DB Standing Shoulder Press	4 sets x 10 reps (2010) - rest 60s	
F	DB Preacher Hammer Curls (L/R)	3 sets x 10 reps - rest 60s	
G	DB Overhead Triceps Extensions	3 sets x 10 reps (3010) - rest 60s	
WK8-D3	same as WK8-D1	replace Pull-Ups with Chin-Ups	
WK8-D4	same as WK8-D2		

GLOSSARY

A, B, C: Exercise-routine labeling format in which each letter denotes a specific exercise (its sets and reps) to be completed before moving on to the next letter. E.g.: Complete Exercise A before moving on to Exercise B. Complete Exercise B, and then move on to Exercise C.

A1, A2, A3: Exercise-routine labeling format in which each letter and number denote a specific exercise (its sets and reps) to be completed before moving on to the next letter and number. E.g.: Complete Exercise A1, A2, and A3 for the specified number of sets and reps, and then move on to Exercise B.

AMRAP: As many reps as possible.

BB: Barbell.

BODY ENGLISH: A movement of the body in an unusual way to create momentum to influence the lift rather than using proper form, e.g., cheating the weight up by using your hips or swinging the weights.

BUILD-UP: The gradual increase of resistance per set toward working sets. They are the warm-up sets that prepare you for the heavier or challenging sets.

BW: Bodyweight.

CIRCUIT TRAINING: A style of training in which two or more exercises are done in succession, with little or no rest between the exercises. The rest occurs after all exercises are completed. The circuit is then repeated.

COMPOUND MOVEMENT: An exercise that involves multiple muscles and the movement of multiple joints, e.g., A bench press involves chest, triceps, shoulder muscles, and joint movement of the elbows and shoulders.

COMPOUND SET: Performing two exercises of the same muscle group with little or no rest, e.g., performing a bench press and then performing dumbbell chest presses, and repeating that sequence for a specified number of sets.

CONCENTRIC: The part of the exercise when the muscle contracts most. Also known as the positive component of the exercise or the lifting phase.

DB: Dumbbell.

DEAD STOP: The lifting technique that eliminates momentum or bounce from the lift by resting the barbell or weight "dead" on the floor, e.g., Deadlifts and Pendlay Rows.

DIRTY 30S: A set of reps in which ten reps are performed in the top half, ten reps in the bottom half, and ten in the full movement of the exercise.

DROP SET: Multiple sets are performed in descending resistance or reduced by specified percentage or weight drops. Can be performed based on failure reps or specific reps. Usually performed at the end of a set.

ECCENTRIC: The part of the exercise in which the muscle stretches most. Also known as the negative component of the exercise or the lowering phase.

ENDURANCE: Muscular endurance is the ability of the muscles to do work against resistance for an extended period of time, e.g., higher-volume sets and reps, high-rep bodyweight exercises, or long-distance running.

FAILURE: The point at which it is impossible to perform an exercise any longer because of muscular failure or fatigue.

GIANT SET: Performing exercises of the same muscle group with little or no rest, e.g., performing a bench press, dumbbell chest presses, and dumbbell chest flyes, and then repeating that sequence for a specified number of sets.

HYPERTROPHY: The increase and growth of muscle.

ISOLATION MOVEMENT: An exercise that involves a single muscle and the movement of one joint, e.g., leg extensions involve quads and the movement of the knee joint.

ISOMETRIC: The holding or pausing of an exercise. Can occur at full contraction.

KB: Kettlebell.

L/R: Left/right. Perform the exercise for the left side and then the right side, or right and then left.

MB: Medicine Ball.

NEGATIVE: The eccentric part of the exercise in which the muscles are most stretched. The lowering of weight with gravity.

POSITIVE: The concentric part of the exercise in which the muscles are contracted. The lifting or raising of weight against gravity.

POWER: Strength x speed. The explosive display of strength.

PR: Personal record. The maximum weight one has lifted on a specific lift.

PROGRESSION: A more difficult version of the exercise.

PYRAMID DOWN: Multiple sets are performed with descending (increasingly light) resistance.

PYRAMID UP: Multiple sets are performed with ascending (increasingly heavy) resistance.

RACK: The equipment onto which a barbell is rested or loaded, e.g., the squat rack or power rack.

REGRESSION: An easier version of the exercise.

REPS: Repetitions. The number of times one lifts and lowers a weight; the lift-and-lower movement of an exercise; or the complete movement of an exercise.

REST: The time between sets for recovery.

RPE: Rate of perceived exertion. A scale from 1 to 10 of the subjective demand of an exercise, e.g., RPE 7 means the demand of an exercise should be 7 out of 10, or 70% effort.

RUN RACK DOWN: Similar to Pyramid Down, in which sets are performed with descending (increasingly light) resistance and applied to dumbbells. Usually decreasing five to ten pounds per set.

RUN RACK UP: Similar to Pyramid Up, but sets are performed with ascending (increasingly heavy) resistance and applied to dumbbells. Usually increasing five to ten pounds per set.

S: Seconds of time. Used for denoting rest intervals between sets or the tempo of movements.

SETS: A collection of repetitions without rest. The number of times one performs a collection of reps, e.g., with 3 sets x 10 reps, one completes ten reps three times, or ten reps, ten reps, ten reps.

SPEED: The amount of time to complete a movement or movements.

STACK: Abbreviation for the weight stack on cable machines, where pins are used to select resistance.

STRENGTH: The force one produces against an external resistance.

STRIP SET: Similar to Pyramid Down, where sets are performed in descending (increasingly light) resistance and applied to plates (plates are stripped off) or machines (the number of stack plates is reduced).

SUPERSET: Performing two exercises of differing muscle groups with little or no rest, e.g., performing a bench press, then performing pull-ups, and repeating that sequence for a specified number of sets.

TEMPO: The speed at which the exercise is performed in seconds. Also displayed as (2010).

TUT: Time under tension. The technique of slowing down repetitions. The muscle is under tension over a longer period of time.

WARM-UP: The act of performing dynamic stretches or exercises to prepare for a full workout or a series of exercises or demanding lifts. The warm-up can also be lighter-weight sets that prepare for heavier loads.

WOD: Workout of the Day.

WORK CAPACITY: The ability to take in, process, and deliver oxygen to do work. Also known as cardiovascular capacity, cardio, or conditioning.

WORKING SETS: The prescribed work sets, not including warm-up or build-up sets.

WORKOUT: A series of exercises.

X: Standard writing convention for "of" or the multiplier when writing workout routine descriptions, e.g., "3 sets of 4 reps" can be written as "3 sets x 4 reps" or just "3 x 4."

1RM: 1 rep max. The maximum weight one can lift for one repetition of a lift/exercise.

PERCENT 1RM: A percentage of 1 rep max. The maximum weight you can lift for one repetition multiplied by a percentage, e.g., 70% 1RM means if your 1 rep max for a lift is one hundred pounds, then you would lift seventy pounds.

(####): Denotes the tempo of an exercise. The time in seconds to lower the weight (negative/eccentric); the time in seconds to pause at the most stretched position; the time in seconds to lift the weight (positive/concentric); and the time in seconds to pause at peak contraction, e.g., a squat of (4321) means it takes four seconds to lower, with a three-second pause or hold at the bottom, two seconds to lift/squat, and one second to pause or hold at the top.

+: The plus/addition sign means more sets or reps (e.g., 5+ sets = five or more sets) or an increase in weight (e.g., +5 pounds/set = increase another five pounds for every set).

±: Plus or minus the recommended quantity, an estimated range.

ACKNOWLEDGMENTS

I want to thank my family and friends for their unconditional support. Thank you to my past clients whom I have trained and to class participants who entrusted me with their fitness guidance. A special thank-you to my training partners throughout the years. We did hard work and had too many laughs. A thank-you to my online fans who share my fitness passion and who constantly inspire and motivate me. Without all your support, I wouldn't have been able to create my artwork or this book. I am humbled and thankful.